Clinical Governance

A Guide to Implementation for Healthcare Professionals

Third Edition

Rob McSherry
Professor of Nursing and Practice Development
School of Health and Social Care,
Teesside University, Middlesborough

and

Paddy Pearce
Assistant Director of Governance
NHS North Yorkshire and York, Thirsk, North Yorkshire

with a contribution by

John Tingle
BA (Law Hons), MEd, Barrister
Reader in Health Law
Director of the Centre for Health Law
Nottingham Trent University, Nottingham

WILEY-BLACKWELL
A John Wiley & Sons, Ltd., Publication

This edition first published 2011
First edition published 2002 by Blackwell Publishing Ltd
Second edition published 2007 by Blackwell Publishing Ltd

Blackwell Publishing was acquired by John Wiley & Sons in February 2007. Blackwell's publishing programme has been merged with Wiley's global Scientific, Technical, and Medical business to form Wiley-Blackwell.

Registered office
John Wiley & Sons Ltd, The Atrium, Southern Gate, Chichester, West Sussex, PO19 8SQ, United Kingdom

Editorial offices
9600 Garsington Road, Oxford, OX4 2DQ, United Kingdom
2121 State Avenue, Ames, Iowa 50014-8300, USA

For details of our global editorial offices, for customer services and for information about how to apply for permission to reuse the copyright material in this book please see our website at www.wiley.com/wiley-blackwell.

Library of Congress Cataloging-in-Publication Data
McSherry, Robert.
Clinical governance : a guide to implementation for healthcare professionals/Rob McSherry and Paddy Pearce, with a contribution by John Tingle. – 3rd ed.
p.; cm.
Includes bibliographical references and index.
ISBN 978-1-4443-3111-0 (pbk. : alk. paper)
1. Medical care–Quality control. 2. Medical audit. 3. Clinical competence. I. Pearce, Paddy. II. Tingle, John. III. Title.
[DNLM: 1. State Medicine–standards. 2. Clinical Medicine–standards. 3. Medical Audit. 4. Patient Care Management–standards. 5. Quality Assurance, Health Care. W 225 M478 2011]
RA399.A1M375 2011
362.1068–dc22
2010014066

A catalogue record for this book is available from the British Library.

Set in 10/12.5 pt Sabon by Aptara® Inc., New Delhi, India

1 2011

Clinical Governance

A Guide to Implementation for Healthcare Professionals

Third Edition

Dedication

To my late parents Wilfred and Dorothy McSherry who I miss dearly. You are always in my thoughts and would have been proud to share this with me.

Rob McSherry

To Samuel Patrick Avison, my grandson.

Paddy Pearce

Contents

Foreword

The National Health Service today looks very different to the National Health Service of 1948. The early years were filled with optimism. Indeed, the costs of the National Health Service were predicted to fall as the health of the nation improved. The early years were characterised by community spirit and those working in the system believed they were contributing to a great project. The public were tremendously relieved that they would no longer have to forgo health care for lack of money.

Demand grew, costs spiralled and the system reached breaking point. A second era began with a major restructuring in 1982 aiming at simplifying the multi-tiered and fragmented National Health Service structures that had developed. The introduction of general management, performance indicators and the internal market aimed to streamline the service, break up the monolithic bureaucracy and create a responsive, financially accountable organisation.

We have now entered a third era, that of quality. Clinical effectiveness, patient safety and patient experience are to be placed at the centre of everything the National Health Service does. Clinical Governance is an essential part of this project to improve the very nature of the healthcare that is delivered. In helping further understanding of the concept, the factors that affect it and the potential impact it represents, this third edition of Clinical Governance offers a valuable contribution to the work being done to make this improvement. Through the processes of clinical governance, clinicians lead from the heart of the system. The setting of standards, collection of data and continuous quality improvement are the bedrock of the future National Health Service.

In his report on the future of the NHS, *High Quality Care for All*, Lord Darzi wrote of quality as being the 'guiding principle'. When I formulated the concept of clinical governance ten years ago, this was a dream. Today it is becoming reality.

Professor Sir Liam Donaldson
Chief Medical Officer
Department of Health

Preface

We are delighted to present this third edition of *Clinical Governance: A Guide to Implementation for Healthcare Professionals*. In this edition we have retained many of the key features of the original text particularly with regard to:

- The evolution of clinical governance
- What clinical governance is
- What the key components of clinical governance are
- The legal implications of clinical governance
- The barriers to implementing clinical governance in clinical practice
- The impact of clinical governance

In this edition we have developed the original theme of healthcare governance towards a more integrated approach to achieving clinical governance with the additional chapter on Education and training for clinical governance. Yet again in this edition we aim to answer the above by using reflective questions, activities and case studies taken within today's healthcare services. The information contained in the book is based upon a combination of the authors' clinical experiences, knowledge and understanding of 'clinical governance an integrated approach' derived from reading and reviewing the associated literature.

Rob McSherry
Paddy Pearce

Chapter 1

Introduction and Background: Clinical Governance and the National Health Service

Rob McSherry and Paddy Pearce

Introduction

This chapter briefly describes the term 'clinical governance', identifying the key drivers for its inauguration into the National Health Service (NHS). The term 'clinical governance' became prominent following the publication of New Labour's first White Paper on health, *The New NHS Modern and Dependable* (Department of Health 1997). Within this document the government sets out its agenda of modernising the NHS by focusing on quality improvements. Clinical quality is rightfully assigned centre stage by 'placing duties and expectation on local healthcare organizations as well as individuals' (DH 1997, p. 34) to provide clinical excellence. The vehicle for delivering clinical quality is termed 'clinical governance', which 'is being put in place in order to tackle the wide differences in quality of care throughout the country, as well as helping to address public concern about well-published cases of poor professional performance' (King's Fund 1999, p. 1). We believe that a complicated series of multiple factors have contributed to the development of clinical governance agenda within healthcare. These can be distilled and categorised into three main drivers: political, professional and public demands, all attempting to revive a failing NHS and improve the quality of care that the public should rightfully expect in a modern society (McSherry 2004).

Clinical Governance, third edition. By Rob McSherry and Paddy Pearce.

Background

Why the need for clinical governance?

The literature offered by Scally and Donaldson (1998), Harvey (1998) and Swage (1998) attributes the need for clinical governance because of a decline in the standards and quality of healthcare provision, a point reinforced by the government. 'A series of well publicized lapses in quality have prompted doubts in the minds of patients about the overall standard of care they may receive' (DH 1997, p. 5). Upon reviewing the early literature (Donaldson & Halligan 2001) on clinical governance we have noted that a key question had not been fully addressed in establishing why there was a perception in the decline of standards and quality. Possible reasons for this perception could be attributed to the following. Firstly, healthcare professionals and the public are better informed and educated and are interested in health-related issues, thus demanding high quality service provision. Secondly, quality and clinical standards have taken a back seat to other financial and resource management issues. Thirdly, political and societal changes have led to a consumerist society where patients and their carers expect to choose where and when they access healthcare. Fourthly, high quality care is seen as a prerequisite. Within this chapter it is our intention to explore the factors that may have contributed to the introduction of clinical governance.

Activity 1.1 Reflective question.

Write down the factors that you feel may have led to the introduction of clinical governance.

Read on and compare your answers with the findings at the end of the chapter.

No single factor has and transformation led to the government's current position for modernisation, reform. We argue that patients' and carers' expectations and demands of all healthcare professionals have significantly increased over the past decade. In the 1980s and early 1990s, public awareness of healthcare provision was increased through target facilitation by the publication of significant documents; notably, *The Patient's Charter* (DH 1992) and *The Citizen's Charter* (DH 1993) both of which were readily and freely made available to the public. On the one hand, these charters may have increased patients' and carers' expectations of healthcare by offering information about certain rights to care. On the other hand, the responsibilities of the patients to use these rights in a responsible way have been over used, resulting in higher demands for care and services in an already busy organisation. Between 1990s and 2005, we have seen a huge emphasis placed on patient and public involvement (PPI) in the planning, delivery and quality assessment of care. Public and patient involvement has been targeted at both a national and a local level both directly and indirectly through the establishment of Patient Advisory and Liaison Services (PALS; DH 2000a) within every NHS organisations. Nationally, we have witnessed the establishment of the Commission for Patient and Public Involvement (DH 2003) resulting in the creation of Patient and Public User Involvement Fora. Similarly, the development of the Overview and Scrutiny Committees for Health (HMSO 2002) with the sole purpose of seeking and representing public opinion on the quality of healthcare. Between 2008 and 2009, further reforms have been introduced surrounding patient and public involvement. We have seen the demise of Patient and Public Involvement Fora and the introduction of Local Involvement Networks (LINks; DH 2008a) which embraces a joined up approach to patient, client, carer and/or user involvement within health and social care and local government. The aim of LINks as defined by the DH (2008a, p. 1) is

> to give citizens a stronger voice in how their health and social care services are delivered. Run by local individuals and groups and independently supported – the role of LINks is to find out what people want, monitor local services and to use their powers to hold them to account.

In addition, other contributing factors such as changes in health policy, demographic changes, increased patient dependency, changes in healthcare delivery systems, trends towards greater access to healthcare information, advances in health technology, increased media coverage of health care and rising numbers of complaints going to litigation have influenced the need for a unified approach to providing and assuring clinical quality via clinical governance (Mc Neil 1998). These will now be debated in further detail under three broad headings and associated subheadings (Fig. 1.1).

Political

Political drivers for governance should be viewed with both a capital and a small 'p'. The capital 'P' refers to those drivers resulting directly from government and policy. The small 'p' relates to organisation and personal factors that influence change and policy decision-making at a local level, a view held by Jarrold (2005)

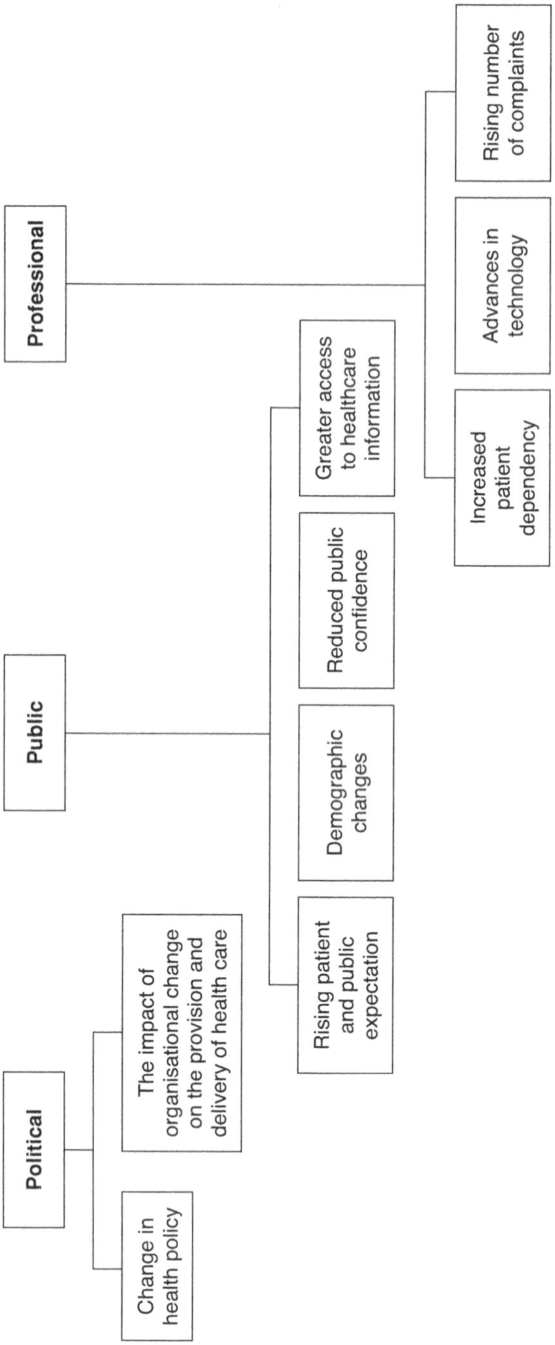

Fig. 1.1 The drivers of clinical governance.

> politics with a small p makes the world go round. Getting things done, seeking support, building alliances, compromising – that's all politics, and inescapable and natural. (p. 35)

The challenge for healthcare professionals is translating policy into practice and keeping up-to-date with changes in healthcare policy.

Changes in health policy

In brief, the NHS was established in 1948 following the passing of the National Health Services Act 1946 which committed the government at the time to financially funding the health service 'which rested on the principles of collectivism, comprehensiveness, equality and universality' (Allsop 1986, p. 12. The politicians at the time thought that by addressing the healthcare needs of the public, this would subsequently reduce the amount of money required to maintain the NHS. The assumption being that disease could be controlled. However, this was not the case. The NHS activity spiralled, resulting in uncontrollable year-on-year expenditures to meet the rise in public demand for healthcare. In an attempt to manage this trend, the government introduced the principles of general management into the NHS (Griffiths Report 1983). The philosophy of general management was concerned with developing efficiency and effectiveness of services. The rationale behind this report was to provide services that addressed healthcare needs (effectiveness) within optimal resource allocation (efficiency). It recommended

> that general managers should be appointed at all levels in the NHS to provide leadership, introduce a continual search for change and cost improvement, motivate staff and develop a more dynamic management approach. (Ham 1986, p. 33)

Key organisational processes identified as missing in the report.

> Absence of this general management support means that there is no driving force seeking and accepting direct and personal responsibility for developing management plans, securing their implementation and monitoring actual achievement. It means that the process of devolution of responsibility, including discharging responsibility to units, is far too slow. (Griffiths Report 1983, p. 12)

This approach, whilst noble at the time, was concerned with organisational, managerial and financial aspects of the NHS, to the detriment of other important issues such as clinical quality. This style of management further evolved with the introduction of the White Paper *Working for Patients* (1989), culminating in the development of a 'market forces' approach to the organisation and delivery of the healthcare services by the creation of a purchaser and provider spilt. Health authorities and general practitioner fund holders were allocated resources (finances) to purchase care for their local population at the best price. It appears that the purchaser/provider split 'did nothing more than engender a lack of strategic coordination between healthcare agencies, as they were encouraged to meet their own financial agendas rather than work in partnership' (Wilkinson 1999, p. 86) or in the maintenance and development of clinical quality. These imbalances led to the introduction of the White Papers *The New NHS Modern and Dependable* (DH 1997) and *Quality in the New NHS* (DH 1998) putting clinical quality on par with organisational, managerial and financial aspects of health care via 'clinical governance'. A framework 'which is viewed positively by many healthcare professionals as an ambitious shift of focus by the current government in moving away from finance to quality' (McSherry & Haddock 1999, p. 114). This approach to providing healthcare services places a statutory duty to match moral responsibilities and harmonises managers and clinicians responsibilities/duties more closely in assuring clinical and non-clinical quality. The impact of these reforms (DH 1989, 1997, 1998a) has enhanced public awareness and expectations for NHS as it places a strong emphasis on achieving clinical quality through restructuring and changing of services.

The DH continued drive for quality improvement through governance and PPI has seen further initiatives introduced by National Health Service Foundation Trusts (DH 2009a), which are 'a new type of NHS organization, established as independent, not-for-profit public benefit corporations with accountability to their local communities rather than Central Government control ... [NHS Foundation Trust] give more power and a greater voice to their local communities and front line staff over the delivery and development of local healthcare. NHS Foundation Trusts have members drawn from patients, the public and staff and are governed by a Board of Governors comprising people elected from and by the membership base' (DH 2009a, p. 1). Creating a patient-led NHS (2005) focused on building the NHS capability and capacity for excellence. Commissioning a patient-led NHS (DH 2005) builds on creating a patient-led NHS by emphasising the importance of efficient and effective commissioning of high quality care. World Class Commissioning (DH 2008a) focused a much needed attention on assuring that commissioning of services reflects the unique needs of each local population whilst seeking to embed a consistent set of performance indicators and patient-related outcomes that demonstrate improvement and comparability of services received across the NHS in England. These recent initiatives seek to increase efficiency and effectiveness and greater PPI at a local level which again have been further consolidated through the publication of *High Quality Care for*

All (DH 2008a) commonly known as the Darzi Report. The essence of the report is as follows:

> Of an NHS that gives patients and the public more information and choice, works in partnership and has quality of care at its heart – quality defined as clinically effective, personal and safe. It will see the NHS deliver high quality care for all users of services in all aspects, not just some. (DH 2008a, p. 8)

Overall, the emphasis of recent government policy (DH 2005, 2008a) has been about increasing the quality of care through seeking out, listening too and responding too the public, health professionals and users of the service(s) by establishing robust systems and processes which demonstrate enhanced patient safety, patient, public and professional involvement, and quality improvement. Furthermore, there is an expectation that has a result of recent reform, patient experience will be improved through having patient-related outcomes that highlights the overall efficiency and effectiveness service.

The impact of organisational change on the provision and delivery of healthcare

With the increases in the numbers of patients admitted with multiple needs, healthcare organisations have had to change the pattern of care delivery in order to accommodate these growing needs, leading to the development of acute medical and surgical assessment units, pre-operative assessment units, multiple needs and rehabilitation units, acute mental health assessment units. Latterly, we have witnessed a rise in the development of services dedicated to maintain individuals in the community, such as Mental Health Crisis Intervention Teams (DH 2001) and the management of patients with long-term conditions, for example diabetes and chronic obstructive pulmonary disease, Fast Response Teams (FRT) such as those jointly provided by Health and Social Care in Harrogate. FRT are designed 'to prevent avoidable hospital admissions, facilitate early discharge and provide out of hours skilled nursing care, thus enabling service users to maintain an optimum level of independence within their own home or care setting' (Care Services Improvement Partnership (Care Services Improvement Partnership Health and Social Care Change Agent Team 2009, p. 1)). This style of service provision is about maximising the use of acute and community beds by encouraging collaborative working between primary and secondary care in the management and maintenance of the patient in the most appropriate setting. For example, in the shared care approach to the management of patients who have diabetes, where the care is shared between the general practitioner and consultant endocrinologist with the backing of the diabetic team (diabetes nurse specialist, dietitian, podiatrist, ophthalmologist and pharmacist). Initiatives such as hospital-at-home schemes (where possible maintaining the patient in their own home) are beginning to be developed along with public and private sector partnerships (acute illness is managed in hospital, and rehabilitation is continued in private nursing home until the patient is ready for discharge).

The driving force behind these innovations could be attributed to the following. The reduction in junior doctors' hours (DH 1998b) and the possible effects of the European working time directive (DH 2004), culminating in the development of nurse practitioners particularly in highly busy areas such as acute medical admissions and accident and emergency departments. This concept was reinforced recently by the introduction of nurse consultants and therapists (McSherry & Johnson 2005) and by the national education and competence framework for advanced critical care practitioners (DH 2008b) in order to accommodate the increasing demands for healthcare owing to the increase in the life expectancy of people with greater healthcare needs. These changes to healthcare delivery are directed towards enhancing the quality of care and in raising public confidence.

Public

The public has contributed significantly towards the introduction of clinical governance and the ongoing development through direct and indirect ways. These vary in nature from rising expectation to changes in demography.

Rising patient and public expectations and involvement

The Patient's Charter (1992) *Raising the Standards* was distributed to all householders in the United Kingdom (UK) detailing the patients' and carers' rights of healthcare. The main principles behind this charter were that of informing and empowering the patients and this led to patients being viewed as consumers of healthcare. As consumers, they are entitled to certain rights and standards of care. These standards included the right to be registered with a general practitioner, to have a named consultant and qualified nurse as an in-patient along with the right to be seen within 30 minutes of any specified appointment time with a healthcare practitioner. The Patient's Charter reinforced the aims of Citizen's Charter (DH 1993) by empowering the individual to become actively involved in the delivery of health services by the granting of certain rights. This style of healthcare delivery was unique, as previously, patients tended to be seen as passive recipients of often-paternalistic methods (the 'doctor knows best') of providing care. The benefits of these charters have been variable, by the fact that some individuals (both the public and healthcare professionals) are unaware of how they can be used to promote raised standards. Alternatively, many patients/carers are much more aware and informed of certain rights to treatments and healthcare interventions. In general, the majority of healthcare professionals have taken up and accepted the challenges posed by these charters in improving the delivery and organisation of healthcare. This can be evidenced by reviewing outpatient waiting time results, hospital league tables and the introduction of the named qualified nurse within inpatient settings. It could be argued that the Patient's Charter has led to a public that are more questioning about their rights and expectations of healthcare: What is the problem? How will the condition be treated? What are the alternatives? What are the potential risks and benefits of all treatment options? These are genuine concerns for the public that need addressing.

While raising awareness and expectations of healthcare services has had a benefit, a limitation of the Patient's Charter is that it has also created a demand which at times has been difficult to satisfy for healthcare trusts. For example, to have a named qualified nurse assess, plan, implement and evaluate care from admission to discharge was impractical and overestimated. Similarly, it is sometimes difficult for a consultant to see all his or her outpatient attendees personally on every visit. The consequence of raising expectations, which are not achievable, results in dissatisfaction with services and higher incidents of complaints. The principles behind the charters are plausible providing the services are resourced sufficiently. Furthermore, the publication of waiting times and league tables has highlighted inequalities in the provision of health care by demonstrating good and poor performers of services. For example, access to services for day case surgery could be variable according to region or demographic status of the local population and geography.

League tables alone do not provide the public with the background information of the local community health trends or the availability of healthcare services for individual trusts, hence the disparity of service provision between trusts. It could be the case that it may be inappropriate to perform day case surgery for hernia repairs in a hospital situated in a rural area with a large elderly population because accessibility of services and appropriateness of the surgery to the patients' needs. This is more evident in society today with an ever increasing elderly population with multi-complex physical, social and psychological needs, placing yet further demands on the health service, making the Patient's Charter standards more difficult to achieve.

Since the introduction of clinical governance through the White Paper (DH 1997) we have seen a dramatic shift from limited PPI to an almost statutory requirement. NHS organisations are systematically required to involve the patients and users in making decisions about the development, provision and experience of the services they have accessed. The Patient and Public Fora (DH 2003) and PALS were two national examples of the government's commitment to improving services for the patients and the public. A key development of PPI has the replacement of Patient and Public Fora with the establishment of LINks in each local authority to actively seek the engagement of patient, public and service users in health and social care. Another imitative exemplifying the government's commitment to patient involvement is the establishment of the NHS Choices Website (NHS 2009) providing accessible information about where patients may receive care and treatment. The choices initiative offers patients the opportunity of choosing where they may wish to have their inpatient investigations, procedures and treatments. Recently the Health Act (2009) highlighted the importance of patient, public and professional involvement by describing the framework for how the NHS Constitution (DH 2009b) designed to

> set out the principles and values of the NHS, It also sets out in one place the rights and responsibilities of patients and staff, and the NHS pledges to patients and staff.

A key outcome of these changes by the government's health polices is seeking to place the patient(s) and service users at the heart of service development, delivery and evaluation. User, patient and professional involvement is critical in a modern consumerist society in ensuring that local services are truly representative and reflective of patient and public needs of that population. This is important in light of changes in demography and dependency.

Demographic changes

Public health policy and findings from national surveys reiterate the government's publication of the *Health of the Nation* (DH 1991) document, which highlighted that life expectancy (National Statistics 2004), would increase for all along with changes in the patterns of mortality and morbidity, for example, an increased prevalence of diabetes and obesity (Press Association 2005). As a consequence of these demographic changes together with changes in morbidity patterns, the NHS needs to provide more acute, continuing care and primary care services for an increasing elderly population and to take into account the changes in the patterns of disease and illness associated with societal change. In an attempt to reduce healthcare demands, the *Health of the Nation* document set targets for reducing morbidity (disease and disability trends) by concentrating upon health promotion and disease prevention. For example, the reduction of strokes by the active management of high blood pressure (hypertension) and the reduction of deaths attributed to coronary heart disease by promoting healthy eating, exercise and, where necessary, the prescription of 'statins' (cholesterol lowering drugs; DH 2000b). The general population changes indicate there has and will continue to be a large increase in the numbers of people living to and beyond sixty-five, seventy-five and eighty-five. Longevity seems to be on the increase for all DH (1991), reinforcing the growing trends of high-dependency patients. Longevity is not the only demographic challenge facing the future NHS; we have seen widening inequalities in health, wealth and disease. There is growing public health concern about obesity, sexual health, drug- and alcohol-related problems, all which will lead to greater demands on the health service and its employees.

Lack of public confidence in healthcare provision due to media coverage of poor clinical practices

The media continues to play a major role in increasing patients' and carers' awareness of the NHS and social care through the publication of clinical successes and failures in the organisations, for example The Bristol case (The Royal Bristol Infirmary Inquiry 2001) and the Shipman Inquiry (The Shipman Inquiry 2005). The Bristol case related to consultant paediatric cardiac surgeons who were found to have a death-rate for paediatric heart surgery significantly higher than the national average. This only became known as a result of whistle blowing (Lancet 1998). The Shipman case involved a general practitioner in Hyde, Manchester, who was found to have murdered hundreds of his patients mainly by injecting them with an overdose of class A drugs such as morphine and diamorphine. The focus on health and social care failings continues to attract growing media attention. The publication of Care Quality Commission (CQC) 'Review of the involvement and action taken by health bodies in relation to the case of Baby P' (CQC 2009) details failings of child protection agencies across health and social care. Similarly, the Healthcare Commission Report 'Investigation into outbreaks of *Clostridium difficile* at Maidstone and Tunbridge Wells NHS Trust' (HCC 2007) highlighted inadequacies with healthcare-associated infection policies and procedures and governance arrangements resulting in increased mortality figures.

The continued impact of these major failings and others has resulted in a lack of public confidence in the health service with a rise in the numbers of complaints proceeding to litigation (Wilson & Tingle 1999).

Trend towards greater access to healthcare information

Advances in information technology, for example the internet have resulted in an easier access to information by the public. Individuals are able to access the same information as healthcare professionals, for example The Cochrane Library and the Department of Health website empowering and informing the public with specific information relating to their condition. This ability to access information, which was perhaps difficult to obtain, previously is fuelling the public's demands and expectations for quality care. Healthcare professionals need to be aware of these rising expectations along with the Freedom of Information Act (DH 2003), which has made access to healthcare information easier. Furthermore, websites such as Doctor Foster (www.drfoster.co.uk) and the National Electronic Library for Health (NeLH) (www.nelh.nhs.uk) reinforce the need for professionals to be aware of giving, receiving and signposting patients and carers to the relevant sources of information. Healthcare professionals also need to be aware of other important factors that may impact on accessing and sharing information such as increased patient dependency and advanced technology.

Professional

Several factors are emerging that may impact on or compromise healthcare professions' accountability. These are associated with increased patient dependency, advanced technology and the rise in litigious activities.

Increased patient dependency

The increasing number of an aging population means that patients are being admitted into acute and community hospitals with far more multi-complex physical, psychological and social problems (McSherry 1999) than ever before, requiring timely appropriate interventions from a wide range of health and social care practitioners. For example, the average length of stay in acute hospital following total hip replacement surgery is around 7 days compared to 14 days, attributed to multi-disciplinary and cross agency collaborative working. A further example is in the advances in stroke care and rehabilitation and in the establishment of specialist stroke units where the evidence (Stroke Unit Trialists' Collaboration 2007) clearly demonstrates that recovery is better if these patients are managed in a specialist unit and not on acute general medical ward. The major effect of rises in dependency levels has resulted in the need for greater efficiency, for example in maximising length of stay and maintaining high levels of acute bed occupancy. However, the shorter average length of patient stay seems to suggest that effective discharge planning is lessened due to staff having less planning time (particularly in complex social cases). Re-admission rates may have increased and certainly higher and greater demands are being made on the community nursing services, hospital-at-home schemes, continuing and long-term care facilitates, as more patients with complex physical and social needs require continued healthcare.

Advances in healthcare designs technology

Advances in healthcare designs technology have made inroads in improving the quality and standards of nursing care delivery, for example pressure relieving equipment, moving and handling equipment, medical administration and monitoring equipment and wound care management. All having the potential for enhancing the quality of care delivered by healthcare professionals. However, credentialisation (demonstrating the evidence that staff have the knowledge, competence and skills to use the equipment safely) may be questionable. The downside is allowing the staff time and resources for education and training to use the equipment in an ever demanding and stressful clinical environment. The latter should not be the case if clinical governance is implemented successfully. These identified pressures being placed upon healthcare professionals to deliver a high quality service based upon appropriate evidence have the potential to create a conflict between balancing efficiency, effectiveness and maintaining quality and standards. These aspirations cannot be achieved for all patients and carers without adequate resourcing and government backing and by some cultural changing.

Rising numbers of complaints going to litigation

Over the past decade there has been a huge rise in the number of formal complaints made by patients and carers about hospital and community services proceeding to litigation. The National Heath Service Litigation Authority (NHSLA) statistics demonstrate rising trends in the number of claims and the total value of claims made between 2003/2004 and 2007/2008 of around £470 million (NHSLA 2005). These rising trends could be attributed to

- Increased activity levels of healthcare
- Greater complexity in treatments and interventions culminating in higher risks associated with increased morbidity
- Greater propensity to pursue and complaint to litigation

- Increased compensations for negligence claims (more likely to seek redress when something goes wrong) if outcome the can result in Monterey gain

It is worth noting here that the vast majority of complaints are resolved at a local level, often with clarification, explanations and the occasional apology for when things have gone wrong. Honesty and openness are the key principles to deal with complaints, as well as developing robust mechanisms for the sharing of information to deal issues before they become problems (McSherry 1996). Management needs to encourage a learning culture, which proactively rather than reactively responds to seek redress when something goes wrong. The ultimate aim is to have a fair blame culture that encourages healthcare professionals to openly report, discuss and learn from clinical incidents or clinical complaints. In many instances, complaints arise from system failures rather than the actions or omissions of individuals. Healthcare professionals need to be made aware of this situation and have the knowledge, skills, competence and confidence to deal positively with complaints.

Summary

Activity 1.1 Feedback.

The contributing factors that lead to and the continuing need for clinical governance can be attributed to the following:

- Changes in health policy
- The impact of organisational change on the commissioning; provision and delivery of healthcare
- Rising patient and public expectations and involvement
- Demographic changes
- Lack of public confidence in healthcare provision due to media coverage of poor clinical practices
- Trend towards greater access to healthcare information
- Increased patient dependency
- Advances in healthcare design technology
- Rising numbers of complaints going to litigation

A closer review of the above factors demonstrates three primary drivers that collectively originate from the 'three p' approach to clinical governance: political, professional and public.

It is clear from Activity 1.1 that there are many contributing factors that influenced the introduction of clinical governance within the NHS. Undoubtedly, more factors will continue to arise reinforcing the need for clinical governance in the future. It is therefore important that organisations and individuals embrace the concept of clinical governance in the pursuit of clinical excellence. The latter can only be achieved by having an understanding of where clinical governance originated and what it means in daily clinical practice as outlined in Chapter 2.

Key points

- The reason for introducing clinical governance into the NHS was a perceived decline in clinical standard, service provision and delivery. This was reinforced by media coverage of major clinical failures notably the Bristol case and the Shipman inquiry resulting a general lack of public confidence in their NHS.
- A more informed consumer-orientated public with greater expectations of the NHS attributed to the different charters.
- A more questioning and litigious society.
- A combination of political, professional and public factors lead to the introduction of clinical governance and the pursuit for quality in the NHS.
- Greater and easier access to information.

Suggested reading

Donaldson, L.J. & Muir Grey, J.A. (1998) Clinical governance: a quality duty for health organizations. *Quality in Healthcare*, 7 (Suppl.) S37–S44.

Mc Neil, J. (1998) Clinical governance: the whys, whats, and hows for theatre practitioners. *British Journal of Theatre Nursing*, 9 (5) 208–216.

Pickering, S. & Thompson, J. (2003) *Clinical Governance and Best Value: Meeting the Modernization Agenda*. Churchill Livingstone, London.

References

Allsop, J. (1986) *Health Policy and the National Health Service*. Longman, London.

Care Services Improvement Partnership Health and Social Care Change Agent Team (2009) *Harrogate Fast Response Team*. http://www.changeagentteam.org.uk/index.cfm?pid=69&catalogueContentID=86. Accessed 2 June 2009.

Department of Health (1989) *White Paper: Working for Patients*. HMSO, London.

Department of Health (1991) *Health of the Nation*. HMSO, London.

Department of Health (1992) *Raising the Standards*. HMSO, London.
Department of Health (1993) *The Citizen's Charter*. HMSO, London.
Department of Health (1997) *The New NHS Modern and Dependable*. HMSO, London.
Department of Health (1998a) *Quality in the New NHS*. HMSO, London.
Department of Health (1998b) Reducing junior doctors' continuing action to meet new deal standards rest periods and working arrangements, improving catering and accommodation for juniors, other action points. *Health Services Circular 1998/240*. DH, London.
Department of Health (2000a) *The NHS Plan: A Plan for Investment, a Plan for Reform*. HMSO, London.
Department of Health (2000b) *National Service Framework for Coronary Heart Disease: Modern Standards & Service Models*. DH, London.
Department of Health (2003) *Freedom of Information Act 2000*. http://www.dh.gov.uk/PublicationsAndStatistics/FreedomOfInformation/FreedomOfInformationAct2000/fs/en?CONTENT_ID=4055574&chk=KOAYUH.
Department of Health (2001) *Major Cash Boost for Mental Health Services*. http://www.dh.gov.uk/PublicationsAndStatistics/PressReleases/PressReleases-Notices/fs/en?CONTENT_ID=4011514&chk=dUYGu/.
Department of Health (2003) http://www.dh.gov.uk/PublicationsAndStatistics/PressReleases/PressReleasesNotices/fs/en?CONTENT_ID=4062851&chk=/YNcaY.
Department of Health (2004) *European Working Time Directive*. http://www.dh.gov.uk/PolicyAndGuidance/HumanResourcesAndTraining/WorkingDifferently/EuropeanWorkingTimeDirective/fs/en.
Department of Health (2008a) *Local Involvement Networks (LiNks)*. http://www.dh.gov.uk/en/Managingyourorganisation/PatientAndPublicinvolvement/DH_076366. Accessed 2nd June 2009.
Department Health (2008b) *The National Education and Competence Framework for Advanced Critical Care Practitioners*. http://www.dh.gov.uk/en/Publicationsandstatistics/Publications/PublicationsPolicyAndGuidance/DH_084011. Accessed 2nd June 2008.
Department of Health (2009a) *Background to NHS Foundation Trusts*. http://www.dh.gov.uk/en/Healthcare/Secondarycare/NHSfoundationtrust/DH_4062852. Accessed 2nd June 2009.
Department of Health (2009b) *The NHS Constitution*. http://www.dh.gov.uk/nhsconstitution. Accessed 2nd June 2009.
DH (2005) Commissioning a patient lead NHS. DH, London.
DH Health Act (2009) http://www.opsi.gov.uk/acts/acts2009/ukpga_20090021_en_1. Accessed 6 May 2010.
Donaldson, L. & Halligan, A. (2001) Implementing clinical governance: turning vision into reality. *BMJ*, 322 (7299).
Donaldson, L.J. & Muir Grey, J.A. (1998) Clinical governance; a quality duty for health organizations. *Quality in Healthcare*, 7 (Suppl.) S37–S44.
Griffiths, R. (1983) *NHS Management Enquiry*. Department of Health and Social Security, London.
Ham, C. (1986) *Health Policy in Britain*. Macmillan, London.

Harvey, G. (1998) Improving patient care: getting to grips with clinical governance. *RCN Magazine*. Autumn.
HMSO (2002) Statutory Instrument 2002 No. 3048. http://www.opsi.gov.uk/si/si2002/20023048.htm. Accessed 6 May 2010.
Jarrold, K. (2005) Being a better manager. *Health Service Journal*, 8 December, p. 35.
King's Fund (1999) *Briefing; What Is Clinical Governance?* King's Fund, London.
The Lancet (1998) Editorial: first lessons from the 'Bristol Case' *The Lancet* 135, 9117, 1619.
Mc Neil, J. (1998) Clinical governance: the whys, whats, and hows for theatre practitioners. *British Journal of Theatre Nursing*, 9 (5) 208–216.
McSherry, R. (1996) Multidisciplinary approach to patient communication. *Nursing Times*, 92 (8) 42–43.
McSherry, R. (1999) Supporting patients and their families. *Caring for the Seriously Ill Patient* (eds C.C. Bassett & L. Makin). Arnold, London.
McSherry, R (2004) Practice development and health care governance; recipe for modernization. *Journal of Nursing Management* (12) 137–146.
McSherry, R. & Haddock, J. (1999) Evidence based health ca vide the complete details along with year and the re: its place within clinical governance. *British Journal of Nursing*, 8 (2) 113–117.
McSherry, R, Johnson, S (2005) (eds) *Demystifying the Nurse/Therapist Consultant. A Foundation Text*. Nelson Thornes Ltd, Cheltenham.
National Electronic Library for Health (NeLH). http://www.library.nhs.uk/default.aspx. Accessed 6 May 2010.
National Health Service (2009) *NHS Choices: Your Health, Your Choices*. http://www.nhs.uk/Pages/HomePage.aspx. Accessed 2nd June 2009.
National Statistics (2004) http://www.statistics.gov.uk/cci/nugget.asp?id=881.
NHSLA (2005) http://www.nhsla.com/Claims/.
Press Association (2005) Obesity levels continue to rise. *The Guardian*, 16 December.
Scally, G. & Donaldson, L.J. (1998) Clinical governance and the drive for quality improvement in the new NHS in England. *BMJ*, 317, 61–65.
Stroke Unit Trialists' Collaboration (2007) Organised inpatient (stroke unit) care for stroke. *Cochrane Database of Systematic Reviews*, (4) CD000197. DOI: 10.1002/14651858.CD000197.pub2.
Swage, T (1998) Clinical care takes center stage. *Nursing Times*, 94 (14) 40–41.
The Royal Bristol Infirmary Inquiry (2001) www.Bristol Royal Infirmary Inquiry FINAL REPORT PRINT VERSIONS.htm.
The Shipman Inquiry (2005) www.The Shipman Inquiry.htm.
Wilson, J. & Tingle, J. (1999) *Clinical Risk Modification: A Route to Clinical Governance*. Butterworth Heinemann, Oxford.

Chapter 2

What is Clinical Governance?

Rob McSherry and Paddy Pearce

Introduction

In Chapter 1 the contributing factors that led to the introduction of clinical governance were described and discussed. This chapter explores and explains where clinical governance originated, how this concept was introduced into the National Health Service (NHS) and its implications for healthcare professionals, managers, Trust boards and organisations.

The evolution of clinical governance

The term clinical governance can be traced to the White Paper *The New NHS Modern, Dependable* (DH 1997). This document outlines the New Labour government's strategy for the modernisation of the NHS, with clinical governance described as 'a system which is able to demonstrate, in both primary and secondary care, that systems are in place guaranteeing clinical quality improvements at all levels of healthcare provision. Healthcare organisations will be accountable for the quality of the services they provide' (McSherry & Haddock 1999, p. 113). In essence, clinical governance, in our opinion, is viewed as the panacea for modernisation of the perceived failing of NHS, as reported in media coverage. Prior to describing what the authors believe and understand to mean by the term clinical governance, a fundamental question requires answering. Where did clinical governance stem from?

Origins of clinical governance

Clinical governance evolved out of the term corporate governance, which originated primarily from the business world associated with the London Stock Exchange. The intention of corporate governance in this instance

Clinical Governance, third edition. By Rob McSherry and Paddy Pearce.
Published 2011 by Blackwell Publishing Ltd.

was to safeguard shareholders' investments and companies' assets, the principle being that of protecting investors and minimising company risks from fraud and malpractice, e.g. the demise of Barings bank as a result of the practices of Nick Leeson (Chua-Eoan 1995). In an attempt to prevent similar incidents within the UK stock exchange, the Cadbury Committee was established. This committee reported in 1992 defining corporate governance as 'the system by which companies are directed and controlled' (NHS Executive 1999). Cadbury identified three fundamental requirements to assure corporate governance within organisations:

- Internal financial controls, i.e. the annual auditing of financial accounts to ensure appropriate use of the company's finances without any underhand dealings.
- Efficient and effective operations, i.e. the company is providing value for money.
- Compliance with laws and regulations, i.e. health and safety is not being compromised; employers and public are protected.

This was termed the 'Cadbury Code'. This code was enhanced by the Greenbury and Hemple Committees, resulting in the publication by the London Stock Exchange of a Combined Code of Principles of Good Governance. The code's major recommendations were that 'the board should maintain a sound system of internal control to safeguard shareholders' investments and company assets': 'The directors should, at least annually, conduct a review of the effectiveness of the group's systems of internal control and should report to the shareholders that they have done so. The review should cover all controls, including financial, operational, and compliance controls and risk management'. (NHS Executive 1999).

Basically this means that corporate governance is about having a systematic approach to demonstrate that the company is doing its best to protect the investors' monies and the company's future, and is complying with statutory obligations. To achieve this, all the company's operational processes require regular monitoring and reviewing in an open and transparent manner.

The Cadbury Code was improved by the Turnbull Committee, which reported in 1999 recommending the need for adequately resourced internal audit departments to evaluate risk and monitor the effectiveness of the company's performance. The potential benefits from corporate governance in the independent sector – open channels of communication, safeguarding public and employees and demonstrating value for money – could equally be applied to the public sector. The government, in an attempt to demonstrate their commitment to improving public service provision, embraced the standards of corporate governance by introducing the principles of corporate governance into the NHS in 1994.

Corporate governance and the NHS

> **Activity 2.1**
>
> How do you think the principles of corporate governance may apply to the NHS?
>
> Read on and then compare your responses with those in the feedback box at the end of this section.

Corporate governance was introduced into the NHS via a three-stage process, which is continuing. This process is described here.

The development of a framework of corporate governance

This was outlined in the publication *Corporate Governance in the NHS; Code of Conduct and Code of Accountability* (NHS Executive 1999), where the focus of the document was directed at NHS Trust boards in ensuring and demonstrating that the conduct of the board was exemplary. The code of conduct for NHS boards is based on three principles shown in Box 2.1.

> **Box 2.1 Principles of corporate governance in the NHS.**
>
> - *Accountability* – everything done by those who work in the NHS must be able to stand the test of parliamentary scrutiny, public judgements on propriety and professional codes of conduct.
> - *Probity* – there should be an absolute standard of honesty in dealing with the assets of the NHS: integrity should be the hallmark of all personal conduct in decisions affecting patients, staff and suppliers, and in the use of information acquired in the course of NHS duties.
> - *Openness* – there should be sufficient transparency about NHS activities to promote confidence between the NHS authority or Trust and its staff, patients and the public.
>
> DH (1994)

Essentially the code of conduct and accountability is about ensuring that each member of staff knows who they are accountable to and for what practices. This should occur in an honest and open environment. Basically this means telling the truth when things go right and when things go wrong.

Improvements in the organisation and staffing of internal audit

This is about ensuring that internal systems are in place throughout the organisation that are working well in highlighting good practice and areas in need of improvement; for example, periodic auditing of staff expenses claims, and vetting the tendering process where external contractors are bidding for NHS work, to gain the best possible quote and ensure value for money.

The development of controls assurance

Controls assurance can be viewed as part of governance and is described as 'a holistic concept based on best governance practice' (NHS Executive 1999, p. 2); that means meeting the codes of conduct, and accountability as previously mentioned. Controls assurance is concerned with methods that enable healthcare organisations to provide evidence that they are doing their 'reasonable best' to manage risk and demonstrate to the public and all stakeholders that they are doing so. Controls assurance is described in more detail later in this chapter. In summary, corporate governance within the NHS is concerned with the non-clinical aspects of healthcare provision that is ensuring financial and operational success by demonstrating value for money. The link to achieve total governance is that of combining the non-clinical with the clinical aspects of healthcare provision. Perhaps this is the primary influence towards the government's introduction of 'clinical governance' within the NHS.

Activity 2.1 ***Feedback.***

Corporate governance is about protecting investors' monies and companies' assets from risks. If these principles are paralleled to the NHS, then corporate governance is about having efficient and effective systems in place to show that money is not being wasted and the services are providing value for money. This is because the NHS is publicly funded via taxation, placing a moral and statutory duty on the management and employees to demonstrate how and where the public money is being spent.

As employees, whether in public or independent sectors, we are governed by contracts of employment, professional regulations and ultimately the civil and criminal laws to provide the best possible services within the given resources. The key word that springs to mind in ensuring corporate governance is accountability. Accountability means that you are able to justify your actions, essentially what you do and why you have to do it.

Defining clinical governance

This section outlines the original definition of clinical governance followed by a review of the working definitions provided by some of the healthcare disciplines. The review compares and contrasts existing definitions culminating in a practical definition by the authors along with identification of the key themes of clinical governance, which are expanded upon in Chapter 3.

The term clinical governance can be traced to the New Labour government's first White Paper on health, *The New NHS Modern, Dependable* (DH 1997) which sets out the government's aims of making the NHS modern and dependable by keeping what has worked in the past and discarding what has failed; for example, the abolition of the internal market that placed finance and activity over clinical quality, leading to fragmentation of services and the ideology of command and control. To resolve these failings the government's philosophy is that of partnerships and collaboration, where innovation is nurtured and staff are valued. The latter is to be achieved by the application of six key principles (see Box 2.2).

Box 2.2 The principles of clinical governance.

1. To re-establish the NHS as a National Service for all patients throughout the country where patients will receive high quality care regardless of age, gender or culture if they are ill or injured.
2. To establish national standards based upon best practices, which will be influenced and delivered locally by the healthcare professionals themselves taking into account the needs of the local population.
3. Collaborative working partnerships between hospital, community services and local authorities, where the patient is the central focus
4. Ensuring that the services are delivering high quality care and providing value for money.
5. To establish an internal culture where clinical quality is guaranteed for all patients.
6. To enhance public confidence in the NHS.

Adapted from DH (1997).

The new structures and systems proposed to achieve the six key principles were a set of national service frameworks (NSFs) (DH 2000a) to be developed with nationally agreed standards, covering major care areas and disease groups, e.g. cancer services, reducing heart disease, mental health and caring for the older person. The purpose of the NSFs is to provide sound equitable and consistent evidence based care and services (DH 2000a, p. 7). Today there are nine NSFs covering the areas of mental health, coronary heart disease, diabetes, renal, older people, cancer, paediatric intensive care, children and long-term conditions. For more detailed information regarding NSFs, visit the NHS Choices website.

A new performance framework with a scorecard of quality effectiveness and efficiency measures, rather than the previous cost and activity focus. This approach to performance management added an important dimension, that of, ensuring clinical care and patient outcome is given equal status to that of finance, cost and activity. The approach has lead to the development of the HCC Annual Health Check, which adopts an even broader review to performance management and is to be implemented by the NHS from 2005. This is discussed in more detail in Chapter 6.

A National Institute for Clinical Excellence (NICE) responsible for the assessment of new technologies and producing robust and authoritative guidelines for the NHS.

A Commission for Health Improvement (CHI). (In 2004 a newly established organisation – the Healthcare Commission for Audit and Inspection – took over from CHI. This organisation is commonly referred to as the Healthcare Commission or HCC.) The purpose of this organisation is to monitor the quality of clinical services at a local level and intervene if necessary to deal with problems and to provide parliament with an annual report on the state of the NHS. In 2009 the HCC merged with the Commission for Social Care Inspection (CSCI) and Mental Health Act Commission (MHAC) to form the Care Quality Commission (CQC). The CQC aims to foster a consistent, collaborative person-centred outcomes based approach to regulation and inspection of health and social care services across the public and independent sectors.

> The Care Quality Commission is the new health and social care regulator for England. We look at the joined up picture of health and social care. Our aim is to ensure better care for everyone in hospital, in a care home and at home (CQC 2009a).

A new system of clinical governance, which is able to demonstrate, in both primary and secondary care, that systems are in place guaranteeing clinical quality improvements at all levels of healthcare provision.

The structures identified above are all individually directed towards establishing and monitoring the level of clinical quality at individual, organisation, region and national levels; for example, The National Institute for Health and Clinical Excellence (previously known as The National Institute for Clinical Excellence (NICE)) continue to set standards and guidelines based on the best available evidence accessible nationally for use by individual health professionals. The role of local NHS Trusts. NHS Foundation Trusts introduced in 2004 '(often referred to as foundation hospitals) are at the cutting edge of the Government's commitment to the decentralisation of public services and the creation of a patient-led NHS. NHS foundation trusts are a new type of NHS trust in England. They have been created to devolve decision-making from central government control to local organisations and communities, so they are more responsive to the needs and wishes of their local people. The introduction of NHS foundation trusts represents a profound change in the history of the NHS and the way in which hospital services are managed and provided' (DH 2009). NHS Foundation Trusts are regulated by 'MONITOR' (MONITOR 2009). MONITOR is an independent regulator of NHS Foundation Trusts. Primary Care Trusts together with Strategic Health Authorities will be to implement these guidelines.

The CQC (has replaced the HCC and CHI) for the regulation and monitoring of healthcare organisations to ensure that these standards are achieved.

Clinical governance according to Donaldson (1998), is viewed as the vehicle to achieve, locally the continuous improvements in clinical quality, that will aid the government's agenda for modernisation of the NHS, evident from the following statement:

> Chief executives will be expected to ensure there are appropriate local arrangements to give them and the NHS Trust board firm assurances that their responsibilities for quality are being met. This might be through the creation of a Board Sub Committee, led by a named senior consultant, nurse, or other clinical professional, with responsibility for ensuring the internal clinical governance of the organisation. (DH 1997, p. 47)

What is clinical governance?

A considerable amount of literature is emerging on the topic of clinical governance, regarding what it is and what it is perceived to be within the various healthcare professions (see Table 2.1).

According to Table 2.1 following the UK government's initial definition of clinical governance the term has become internationally recognised as a whole system/framework for improving quality through minimising risks by embracing patient safety through raising professionals awareness of their own accountability for excellence. The term seems to have been embraced by the majority of healthcare professions. However, some differences emerge in the way individual professions have interpreted, internalised and transferred the meaning of clinical governance for their specific profession. For instance, occupational therapy views clinical governance 'as a framework for combining a full range of quality activities, building first upon what is already being carried out' (Sealey 1999). This definition by Sealey (1999) infers that it is essential to build on existing good practice in a systematic and organised manner. Similarly the Royal College of Nursing (RCN) (1998) defines clinical governance as 'a framework, which helps all clinicians including nurses to continuously

Table 2.1 A critical review of professional perspectives in defining clinical governance.

Author (year)	Professional discipline	Definition	Key themes
DH (1997)	Government	'A framework through which NHS organizations are accountable for continuously improving the quality of their services and safeguarding high standards of care by creating an environment in which excellence in clinical care will flourish'	Framework Accountability Maintaining Improvement Culture Quality Prospering
Sealey (1999)	Occupational therapy	'A framework for combining a full range of quality activities, building first upon what is already being carried out'	Framework Quality Maintaining Improvement
McNeil (1998)	Theatre nursing	'The means by which organizations ensure the provision of quality clinical care by making individuals accountable for setting, maintaining and monitoring performance standards'	Quality Accountability Maintaining Improving Standards Outcome
Scally & Donaldson (1998)	Doctors	'The main vehicle for continuously improving the quality of patient care and developing the capacity of the NHS in England to maintain high standards'	Quality Improvement Maintaining Resource Standards

Table 2.1 *(cont'd)*

Author (year)	Professional discipline	Definition	Key themes
Royal College of Nursing (1998)	Nurses	'A framework which helps all clinicians – including nurses – to continuously improve quality and safeguard standards of care'	Framework Improvement Maintaining Quality Standards Indirectly accountability
World Confederation For Physical Therapy (2000)	Physiotherapist	'A government initiative (introduced in 1998) to provide a framework through which NHS organisations are accountable for continuously improving the quality of services they deliver'	Framework Accountability Quality Improvement
Australian Council of Healthcare Standards (2004)	National	'Clinical governance is the system by which the governing body, managers and clinicians share responsibility and are held accountable for patient care, minimising risks to consumers and for continuously monitoring and improving the quality of clinical care'.	System Accountability Risk management Quality improvement Monitoring

Vaun Som (2004)	Managerial/ organisational	'as a governance system for healthcare organisations that promotes an integrated approach towards management of inputs, structures and processes to improve the outcome of healthcare service delivery where health staff work in an environment of greater accountability for clinical quality'	System Accountability Quality improvement Integration Outcomes
Royal College of General Practitioners (2005)	GP	'The principal aims of clinical governance are to improve the quality and the accountability of healthcare'	Improvement Quality Accountability
Royal Pharmaceutical Society of Great Britain (2005)	Pharmacists	'The means by which organisations ensure the provision of quality clinical care by making individuals accountable for setting, maintaining and monitoring standards'.	Quality Accountability Maintaining Monitoring Standards
NHS Quality Improvement Scotland (2005)	Australian Council of Healthcare Standards	'Clinical governance is the system through which NHS organizations are accountable for continuously monitoring and improving the quality of their care and services and safeguarding high standards of care and services'.	System Accountability Quality improvement Safety Standards

Table 2.1 *(cont'd)*

Author (year)	Professional discipline	Definition	Key themes
Association of Optometrists (2006)	Optometrists	'Has to do with the delivery of high quality clinical services. Clinical governance is to be a welcomed as it makes clinical quality an integral part of the NHS governance framework'	Delivery Quality Framework
British Dental Association (2006)	Dentists	'Is part of the NHS drive to improve the quality of health care and to make providers accountable for delivering a consistent standard on which patients can rely'	Improvement Quality Accountability Delivery Standards
Braithwaite and Travaglia (2008)	Regional	'A systemic and integrated approach to assurance and review of clinical responsibility and accountability that improves quality and safety resulting in optimal patient outcome'.	Integration Assurance Responsibility Accountability Quality Safety Outcomes

improve quality and safeguard standards of care'. The RCN (1998) like Sealey (1999) consider clinical governance as a framework for maintaining, sustaining and improving standards but differs in the way they acknowledge the importance of clinical governance to all professionals groups. A omission of these definitions along with the others provided is the failure to acknowledge and incorporate the contributions from the many non-professional groups like clerical, administration, finance, human resources ancillary, maintenance and engineering staff. There are number of common emergent themes from the definitions offered by the various professional groups with the majority viewing clinical governance as a Department of Health (DH) directive through which individuals and organisation are accountable for clinical quality, service and patient safety. Most definitions acknowledge the fact that clinical governance is a framework that pulls a whole range of organisational departments together by focusing on the systems and processes with a strong emphasis placed on accountability associated with the maintenance and improvement of standards. Clinical governance for us draws together a number of concepts namely:

- The systematic harmonisation of clinical and managerial responsibilities with accountable practice
- Team working and interdependency through integrated working with and between health and social care both public and independent [private]
- Monitoring, changing, evaluating and improving practice to safeguard standards
- The drive for constant quality improvement in all that we do
- Nurturing a culture of continuous learning
- Placing a duty of care to improve individual, team and organisational performance
- Adopting a person-centeredness approach in all that we do is the heart of clinical governance.

The prominent theme from the various definitions is the emphasis on having robust systems/frameworks for ensuring that clinical quality exists throughout the entire organisation, where each individual is accountable for their actions. We would argue that clinical governance could at best be summarised as a robust framework that acknowledges the importance of adopting a culture of shared accountability for sustaining and improving the quality of services and outcomes for both patients and staff. Clinical governance is ultimately 'an umbrella term for all the issues and concepts that clinicians, non-clinicians, mangers and board members know and foster, including standard setting, risk management, patient safety, user involvement, performance management, clinical audit, training, reflection and continuous professional development to name but a few (McSherry & Haddock 1999). Clinical governance is about instilling confidence in both the public and healthcare professionals by providing them with a safe clinical and learning environment in which to accommodate the challenges identified in Chapter 1, which are facing them in the future. In a simple way, clinical governance is about the patients/carers receiving the right care at the right time from the right person in a safe, honest, open and caring environment. To ensure that clinical governance is successfully implemented throughout any healthcare organisation the key components contained within its definition need to be available and achievable throughout the organisation, as the following section will now briefly explain.

The key components of clinical governance

This section introduces the key components of clinical governance and how they relate to individuals, organisations and the wider aspect of the NHS; a more detailed account is offered in Chapter 3.

The definitions of clinical governance identified in Table 2.1 highlight common themes that describe what clinical governance is. These can be summarised into Fig. 2.1.

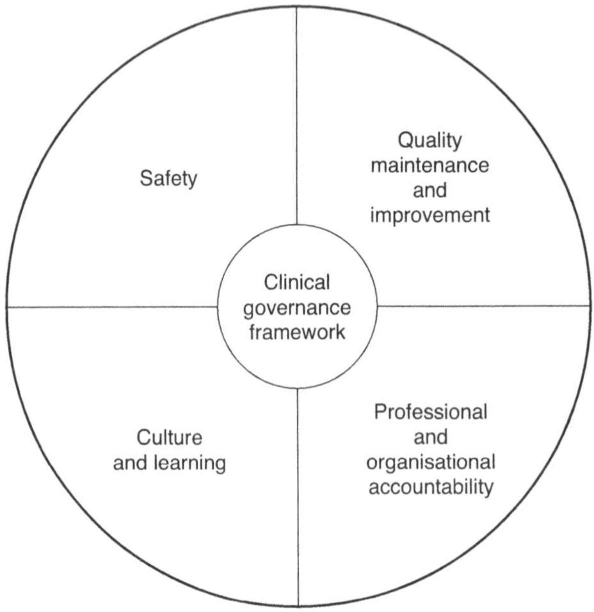

Fig. 2.1 Key components of clinical governance.

Figure 2.1 depicts the key components that make up clinical governance, which in turn could be considered as the building blocks for its success for either an individual or a healthcare organisation. For clinical governance to operate effectively the identified components need to be evident and operational. Clinical quality and continuous improvements in healthcare delivery can only be achieved in a culture and environment which supports, values and develops its staff. Likewise individual healthcare professionals need to continuously develop their professional standards whilst operating within the roles and responsibilities aligned to their contract of employment and codes of professional practice. Essentially clinical governance is about providing good clinical care in an environment, which places patient and staff safety as a number one priority.

It is evident from the above description of the authors' interpretations of the various definitions of clinical governance identified in Table 2.1 that their primary focus is around clinical practices which no one would disagree with, although within these definitions of clinical governance there appear to be no explicit links to the non-clinical aspects of health care which are equally important in proving clinical quality.

Non-clinical services that support clinical governance

Activity 2.2 Non-clinical services that support clinical governance.

List the non-clinical services that support healthcare professionals in executing clinical governance successfully.

Read on and compare your findings with those in the feedback box towards the end of the chapter.

When providing care in a busy and stressful clinical setting it is easy to forget all those other supporting services that are perhaps taken for granted when we provide our services; for example, a simple case of a general practitioner (GP) referring a patient to a consultant for a clinical opinion. This involves the letter from the GP, perhaps dictated for their clerical staff to process, which may be received by the medical records staff or consultant secretaries who in turn arrange an outpatient appointment and inform the patient. The patient subsequently attends the outpatient department to be seen by the consultant. For this to happen effectively, much work is done behind the scenes that involves the following groups of personnel: estate staffs in maintaining the safety of the building and mains services; domestics in maintaining the cleanliness and hygiene standards; and a range of supporting services to enable the operational and clinical staff to perform their duties, such as personnel, finance and information services. Clinical governance cannot be operationalised without the

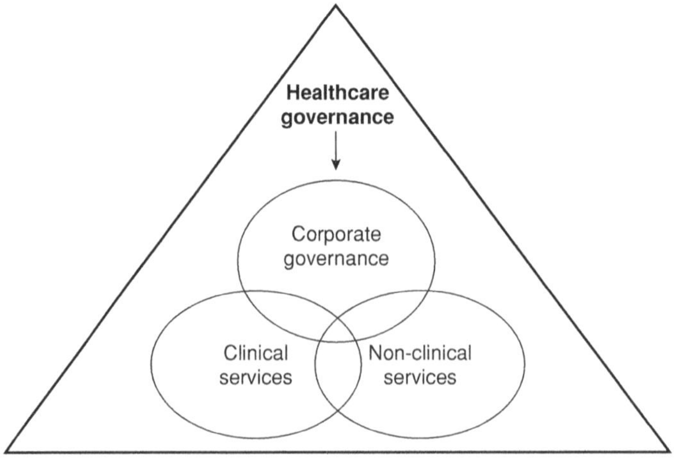

Fig. 2.2 Healthcare governance in the NHS.

non-clinical supporting services, as depicted by the simple example above. This example demonstrates the links between non-clinical supporting activity and clinical governance. Clinical governance cannot be successfully implemented without the support of the non-clinical aspects of healthcare delivery. As most health professionals are fully aware, healthcare provision and delivery is complex in nature. Successful healthcare delivery is dependent on good teamwork, effective leadership and sound management in drawing together the non-clinical and clinical aspects of governance. Basically neither can work effectively without the other, as outlined in Fig. 2.2.

Figure 2.2 highlights the role of healthcare governance in uniting the three elements of health service governance: corporate (management), clinical governance (clinical practice) and the non-clinical supporting services. Whilst there has been much attention directed towards establishing good managerial and clinical practices based on sound evidence in ensuring clinical quality, it would appear that ensuring quality associated with the non-clinical supporting services such as those outlined in Activity 2.2 was not given equal status. To address this imbalance it is important to know that the government initially introduced guidelines and standards for the NHS to assure quality in these parts of the organisation. This was facilitated and achieved through the introduction of 'controls assurance' (NHS Executive 1999).

Controls assurance: Its relationship with clinical governance

When exploring the meaning of clinical governance it is important to remember the role controls assurance played in the developmental processes of measuring compliance with systems and processes deemed necessary to assure quality.

The Health Service Circular 1999/123 describes controls assurance as 'A holistic concept based on best governance practice' (NHS Executive 1999, p. 2). This approach is reinforced and enhanced by Emslie who defines controls assurance as: 'a process, built on best governance practice, by which NHS organisations demonstrate that they are doing their reasonable best to manage themselves so as to meet their objectives and protect patients, staff, visitors, and other stakeholders against risks of all kinds'. (Emslie 2001, p. 1).

The difficulty for many healthcare organisations and individuals is in conceptualising and implementing healthcare governance because they see each component, such as clinical governance, corporate governance and controls assurance, as separate and unrelated entities. The authors accept that many healthcare professionals view the components of healthcare governance in isolation, but we would argue that in practice this is usually not the case. For example, the routine administration of either an intravenous or intramuscular injection involves many clinical and non-clinical healthcare professionals and systems and processes to work efficiently and effectively. Some healthcare professionals only see their part of the overall systems and process(es), such as the preparation and administration. But what happens if the medication and equipment are not available or the 'sharps' are not disposed of safely? This simple illustration demonstrates that healthcare governance is truly a holistic concept that unifies the three components of clinical, non-clinical and corporate governance. Controls assurance is the vehicle that enables each organisation to demonstrate that their systems and processes for assuring healthcare governance are both efficient and effective.

Emslie (2001) provides a model linking corporate (Trust) objectives with providing assurance to their stakeholders of quality healthcare, highlighting the importance of accountability, processes, capability and outcomes, of which each element is continuously monitored and reviewed, and where lessons are learnt, practices improved and risks minimised. Essentially this model can be applied to individuals, teams and organisations. Controls assurance was concerned with methods that enable healthcare organisations to provide evidence that they are doing their 'reasonable best' to manage risk and demonstrate to the public and all stakeholders that they are doing so. The main principle underpinning controls assurance is that of collaborative working, thus ensuring that risks are minimised and where identified are managed appropriately (McSherry & Pearce 2000; Emslie 2001).

Within the Health Service Circular HSC 1999/123 chief executives were advised to appoint an executive director to assume responsibility for the implementation of controls assurance, thus making an individual the accountable officer to parliament. The designated person was charged with reviewing the circular and guidance. Chief executives were responsible for informing the National Controls Assurance Project Manager, who is the designated person for their organisation.

The HSC 1999/123 led to the development of 18 standards covering the non-clinical and some clinical aspects of service delivery, such as infection control, health and safety and waste management. The standards were released on 22 November 1999 at the NHS Controls Assurance Conference which 'forms the basis of a self-assessment exercise to be undertaken by all NHS trusts and health authorities from 2000, leading up to an assurance statement to be signed by chief executives on behalf of boards in their 1999–2000 annual report' (Hopkins 2000, p. 22). In essence controls assurance completed the governance picture by linking the corporate, clinical and non-clinical elements of governance.

More information on controls assurance can be found by reading McSherry and Pearce (2000), NHS Executive (1999) and Hopkins (2000). It is clear from Fig. 2.1 that the key elements of governance all have potential benefits to improve the quality of care that can be further enhanced when these components work in harmony. Since the introduction of the controls assurance standards the NHS has realised the need to adopt an integrated approach to healthcare governance. As a consequence today healthcare governance could be viewed as a Rubik cube incorporating the six faces of governance Fig. 2.3.

According to Fig. 2.3 it is evident that the concept of healthcare governance has evolved incorporating additional elements to those

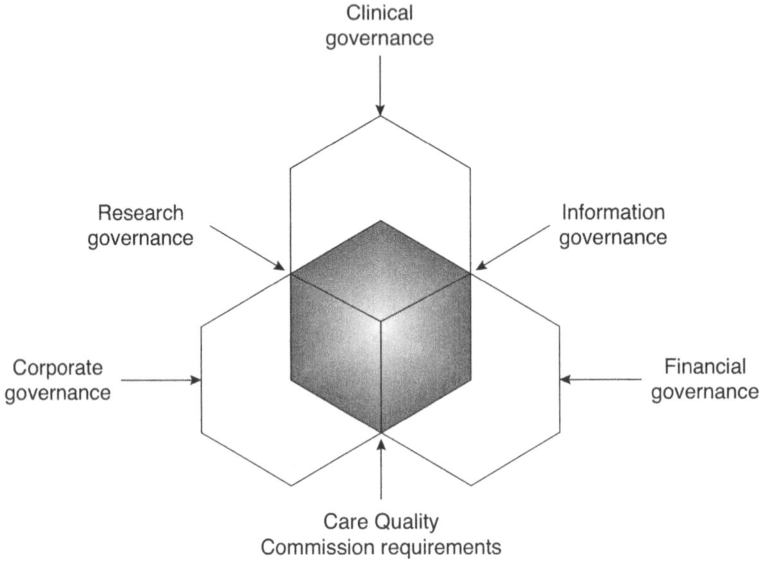

Fig. 2.3 The six faces of healthcare governance.

highlighted previously in Fig. 2.3. Healthcare governance has become a phrase that demonstrates the importance of adopting an intergraded approach to governance in its totality. Healthcare governance today involves clinical governance, information governance, financial governance, care quality requirement commission e.g. registration, corporate governance and research governance. Like the Rubik cube, the benefits can only be fully realised when the six faces of each cube are aligned. Put simply, integrated or healthcare governance is dependent on the efficient and effective alignment and coordination of the various components of governance. Similarly, at an organisational level the various departments that constitute the six faces of the Rubik cube need to cooperate and communicate effectively in an open culture of mutual respect and cooperation. As a consequence of adopting this whole systems approach to governance we have witnessed the demise of controls assurance standards for NHS organisation being replaced with the Standards for Better Health (DH 2004b). These are discussed in the next section.

Standards for better health

The section is replicated with kind permission by the *Healthcare Risk Report*. The information is based upon the works of McSherry & Pearce (2004) titled 'Healthcare standards: a critique of the DH's national standards for the NHS'.

The introduction of the DH's *Standards for Better Health* (DH 2004b) as identified in Chapter 1 can be attributed to a combination of several issues involving societal, political and professional factors. These include changes in health policy, rising patient/carer expectations, increased patient dependency, technology advances, demographic changes in society, changes in care delivery systems, lack of public confidence in the National Health Service (NHS), threat of litigation and demand for greater access to information (McSherry & McSherry 2001).

Activity 2.3

What do you understand by the term national healthcare standards? Why do you think these have been developed? What aspects of health care do you think these standards should cover?

Read on and then compare your responses with those in the feedback box at the end of this section

The need for national healthcare standards

The provision of accessible, equitable, high-quality care and services is difficult for the NHS to achieve. The ideal is a service that provides high-quality services delivered locally by well-trained, motivated people, that delivers the right care to the right individual in the right setting at the right time (McSherry & Pearce 2002, 2007). This approach to service provision must be capable of demonstrating success in a meaningful way to patients, the public and healthcare organisations and ultimately the government.

As highlighted in the previous chapter in recent years a number major clinical and corporate failures in the NHS have attracted adverse media coverage (Smith 1998). The Bristol Royal Infirmary Inquiry found the outcomes and care of children undergoing cardiac surgery there were sub optimal, while the Royal Liverpool Children's Inquiry found that at Alder Hey Children's Hospital, body parts of children were removed and kept without the informed consent of parents. More recently the Mid Staffordshire NHS Foundation Trust was cited by the Healthcare Commission (2009) as a 'story of appalling care and chaotic systems for looking after patients'. Through these examples of major, corporate, organisational and clinical care failures, the public and government have realised that the NHS was and sometimes continues to fail to deliver what the public expects, including clinical outcomes comparable with other western nations. So, what has happened to address service failures and indeed to fulfil the founding aspirational principles of the NHS?

The concept of performance management (detailed in Chapter 3) has been introduced and over the decades the NHS has been subjected to an ever-increasing number of targets and performance measures. A reductionist approach is evident and often what is measured is that which can be counted, such as waiting times in accident and emergency. We would suggest that this approach has been extended to the concept of 'inspection', in this instance referring to internal and external inspection and review to assure the government and the public that the NHS is delivering good quality outcomes.

NHS organisations are reviewed by a diverse range of inspectorates covering a broad spectrum of NHS activity. These inspecting organisations appear to work in splendid isolation, often examining similar areas from a slightly different perspective and on occasion reaching very different conclusions. These inconsistencies lead to confusion over the expectations of the inspectorates, placing ever-increasing demands on NHS organisations, which deploy disproportionate resources into achieving targets and preparing for inspection. The former government's NHS Plan (DH 2000a) promises investment and reform through modernisation. The NHS has undoubtedly been subjected to over inspection with the emphasis on targets leading to low morale and de-motivated staff. This point was highlighted in the Bristol Royal Infirmary Inquiry report and the recommendation made that 'the NHS should have national standards'. In response the DH has attempted to produce national generic standards for the entire service.

Defining the healthcare standards

Healthcare standards in [the Bristol] report are being defined as a level, which others accept as the baseline for good practice, the desired level of achievement (Schroeder & Maibusch 1984). Successive DH White Papers (DH 1997, 1998) place emphasis on the importance of improving and assuring the quality of care, treatment and services through the principles of clinical governance. This is a major feature in guaranteeing quality to the public and the NHS, that clinical, managerial and educational practice is based on measurable evidence (McSherry & Haddock 1999). Quality improvements have been placed at the forefront of the NHS agenda and clinical effectiveness is to be measured and evaluated against the proposed set of healthcare standards.

We would argue that there is a definite need for an integrated approach to the establishment of healthcare standards in the NHS. We would argue this has lead to the establishment of the Care Quality Commission (CQC) which adopts a collaborative integrated approach to reviewing and regulating standards for better health and social care. Organisational standards and accreditation schemes are essential for demonstrating acquired levels of excellence within any organisation. They provide excellent frameworks for promoting quality improvements, and as a result support organisations and professionals in making practice open and accountable. Our recent experiences of working with organisational standards, along with assessing levels of achieved practice, identify that they require organisational and managerial support, resources and financial backing.

Organisational standard measurement is an integral part of quality improvement. Practice areas need to provide evidence to the accrediting bodies to show how they have achieved a particular standard. Bodies such as Care Quality Commission (formerly the Healthcare Commission) and the National Health Service Litigation Authority (NHSLA) through its Clinical Negligence Scheme for Trusts require practice areas to demonstrate how they are providing effective quality care. The difficulties and challenges in the development of healthcare standards are in producing criteria against which they can be easily, consistently and uniformly assessed, which is perhaps a limitation for some existing healthcare standards and accrediting bodies. The way forward to resolving these and many other issues aligned to healthcare standards and accreditation is the production of a generic framework. The government is at least trying to address these issues by consulting with organisations and users of healthcare services on the proposed healthcare standards. The concept of having an integrated set of regulations and standards for which the majority of health and social care providers will have to comply with are provide by the regulation and registration requirements set out by the newly formed CQC. The CQC are responsible for leading the process of regulation and accreditation of health and social care providers in the future. The establishment of the CQC in our opinion was essential to avoid duplication of effort and energy, reduce the burden of inspection on health and social care organisations, to provide an integrated assessment of health and social care across the various health and social care establishments using consistent methodologies and finally to offer assurance to public/users of the service and health and social care professionals themselves about the quality provided.

Describing healthcare standards for better health

The document *Standards for Better Health: Healthcare Standards for Services under the NHS – a consultation* (DH 2004b) was published in February 2004 for a 3-month consultation period. The secretary of state John Reid states in the foreword:

> These standards are not yet another batch of rules and regulations whose object is to tie clinicians into further procedures and targets (DH, 2004b, p. 2).

The document has six key sections, of which section three details 24 core standards, and section four outlines ten developmental standards. These two sections are the key sections with which healthcare organisations and professionals should become familiar. The core standards attempt to set out clearly what patients can expect from the NHS. They do not seek to establish new standards but bring together the vast array of complex and confusing guidelines, measures and assessments. In contrast, developmental standards are not absolute measures but more broad-based, concerned with assessing progress made with implementation of the NHS Plan and other key NHS strategy documents. The challenge for the organisation is in ensuring that they implement and review the core alongside the developmental standards. The 24 core standards are set out within seven domains (Box 2.3).

Box 2.3 Seven domains of healthcare standards.

- Safety
- Clinical and cost effectiveness
- Governance
- Patient focus
- Accessible and responsive care
- Care environment and amenities
- Public health

According to Box 2.1 it would appear that the DH is attempting to provide an integrated approach towards governance. The similarities of the domains with the clinical and corporate governance framework are striking (McSherry & Pearce 2002). But what is behind each of these domains needs further exploration.

Safety is defined as 'the design of healthcare processes, working practices and systematic activities prevent or reduce risk of harm to patients'. There are five associated standards predominately centred on risk, risk management and learning from experience good and not so good. One standard is a developmental standard, about the introduction and enhancement of the systems and processes to monitor and respond to risks continuously.

The definition for clinical and cost effectiveness is that 'health care decisions are based on what appropriately assessed research evidence has shown provides an effective outcome for patients' individual needs'. There are two core standards and one developmental standard. The emphasis is on ensuring that care and treatments are based on best available evidence and guidance.

The definition of governance is that 'all providers of health services have in place the managerial and clinical leadership and accountability, the organisational culture, and the systems and working practices to enable probity, quality assurance, quality improvement and patient safety to be central components of all routines, processes and activities'. This domain is the most comprehensive standards and includes seven core standards and three developmental standards. The emphasis is on integration of clinical and corporate governance frameworks into a holistic and integrated governance model (Deighan *et al.*, 2004).

Patient focus is defined as health care that 'is provided in partnership with patients, their carers and relatives and is designed around decisions which respect their diverse needs, preferences and choices' (DH 2003). The domain includes four core standards and two developmental standards. The central aims of these standards are ensuring equity, equal access to information, the maintenance of confidentiality, and the involvement of carers and patients in their care and treatment and the design/development of new services. By extension we would argue that all of the NHS must be patient-focused.

Accessible and responsive care is identified as patients receiving services promptly as possible, having choice in access to services and treatments, and experiencing the minimum unnecessary delay at any stage of service delivery or the care pathway. The domain contains two core standards and one developmental standard reinforcing the need for healthcare organisations and services to focus their attention on ensuring access and equity of services. It is notable that the patient focus and accessible and responsive care domains go hand in hand and could easily be incorporated as one domain.

Care environment and amenities says that care should be 'provided in environments that promote patient and staff well-being and respect for patients' needs and preferences, in that they are designed for the effective and safe delivery of treatment, care or a specific function (such as catering or pharmacy), accord an appropriate degree of privacy, are well maintained and are cleaned to optimise health outcomes'. This domain includes one core standard and one developmental standard emphasising the need for organisations and individuals to actively consider safety, support, patient privacy and confidentiality. It could be argued that traditionally environmental factors have not been seen as a high priority but are fundamental to patient and staff well-being.

Public health is a new area for standard-setting in the NHS. Public health in this instance is defined as providing 'leadership, and collaborat[ing] with relevant local organisations and communities to ensure the design and delivery of programmes and services which promote, protect and improve the health of the population and reduce inequalities between different population groups and areas'. This is a highly topical and important domain because of changes in demography and society. Furthermore this is an underdeveloped field of practice for many healthcare professionals to implement. The success of this domain depends on developing partnerships and cooperative strategies with other public and commercial enterprises. Primary care trusts should drive this domain forward.

Currently the CQC has published a consultation document 'Guidance about compliance with the Health and Social Care Act 2008 (Registration requirements) regulation 2009 draft guidance' (CQC 2009a). The guidance contains six generic domains comprising 23 regulations (Box 2.4) and 18 specific areas (Box 2.5) covering the full spectrum of health and social care. The proposed guidance on compliance is intended to replace the Department of Health Standards for Better Health (DH 2004b), 'Independent Health Care, National Minimum Standards, Regulations' (DH 2002) and 'National Minimum Standards (CQC 2009b). The proposed new regulations represent a progressive move towards fostering an integrated approach to health and social care delivery across and between public and independent sectors. Furthermore the emphasis is on patient related outcomes as opposed to processes.

Box 2.4 Generic domains.

- Involvement and information
- Personalised care, treatment and support
- Safeguarding and safety
- Suitability of staffing
- Quality and management
- Suitability and management

Box 2.5 Specific regulations.

1. Services provided by an acute hospital, a community hospital, a rehabilitation service, a termination of pregnancy service or a prison health services
2. Services provided by a hospice or a long-term conditions facility
3. Services provided by a mental health or learning disabilities hospital
4. Services provided by a mental health/learning disabilities community service
5. Services provided by a substance misuse rehabilitation and/or treatment service
6. Services provided by an independent doctor
7. Services provided by a community nursing service
8. Services provided by a care home
9. Services provided by a care home with nursing
10. Services provided by a domiciliary care service
11. Services provided by a supported living service
12. Services provided by Shared Lives (formerly known as adult placement)
13. Services provided by a specialist college
14. Services provided by a hyperbaric chamber service
15. Services provided by a diagnostic imaging and/or screening service
16. Services provided by a remote clinical advice service
17. Transport services provided by an NHS provide
18. Services provided by a blood and transplant services

From April 2010 the standards for better health will be replaced with a set of generic registration requirements for all health and social care providers.

The standards versus existing systems

There are several pros and cons that seem to surround the introduction of the previous national healthcare standards for the NHS along with the proposed new regulations for 2010. The concept of a set of national standards and regulation requirements that try to draw together the key components of the business of the NHS and indeed health and social across both independent and public sectors is essential, given the disparity and inequity of service that continue to exist within the NHS, public and independent sectors. NHS, public and independent sector organisations and professionals welcome the introduction of a set of national standards and regulations providing they support professional practice and quality improvement and do not add further to the bureaucracy of existing systems of performance review. However, as the NHS is such a complex and multifaceted organisation is it really possible to introduce such a framework? Previous attempts have resulted in crude measures such as the NHS performance indicators and have led to a lack of confidence in the systems because they were meant to be supportive, proactive and not reactive and policing (McSherry & Pearce 2002). The change in emphasis in developing an integrated patient related outcome focus is a step in the right direction in ensuring a joined up collaborative and partnership working offering the potential of demonstrating the effectiveness of health and social care provision. Furthermore, by having a common generic and specific inclusive set of the regulations may reduce the burden of inspection and the collation of evidence. The HCC and CQC have recognised potential areas were similar areas are assessed and have used the third party evidence as assurance of core standard. For example, some the evidence from The National Health Service Litigation Authority Risk Managements Standards may be used as evidence of compliance with some elements of some generic and specific standards therefore avoiding duplication and burden of evidence gathering and collation.

The challenge to the CQC will be overseeing this process in realising their aspirations of improving health and social care. The challenge for health and social care organisations will be in applying the regulations to existing practice, marrying existing standards of accreditation within the regulations, collecting and collating evidence to demonstrate achievement of compliance with the regulations which could be time consuming, costly and burdensome. Furthermore, will the CQC be able to meet the huge demanding challenge of devising a robust set of methodologies which are reliable, valid and credible to assess that self compliance and disclosures accurately reflect what is happening in reality? Similarly, how will the CQC ensure that these methodologies are rigorously applied fairly, consistently and uniformly across all sectors of health and social care? The key question is: will there be any independent evaluation of the effectiveness of the CQC perhaps this is a role for the Audit Commission or National Audit Office. In essence, how can we ensure to the public that the regulator is been regulated?

Applying the healthcare standards to an example of practice

For the healthcare standards [as with the proposed new regulations (CQC 2009a)] to become an integral part of demonstrable quality in health and social care and improvement, it is fundamental they become adopted and applied at all levels of organisations. To this end a whole systems approach to health and social care governance needs to be developed (McSherry 2004). Figure 2.4 attempts to show how the seven domains

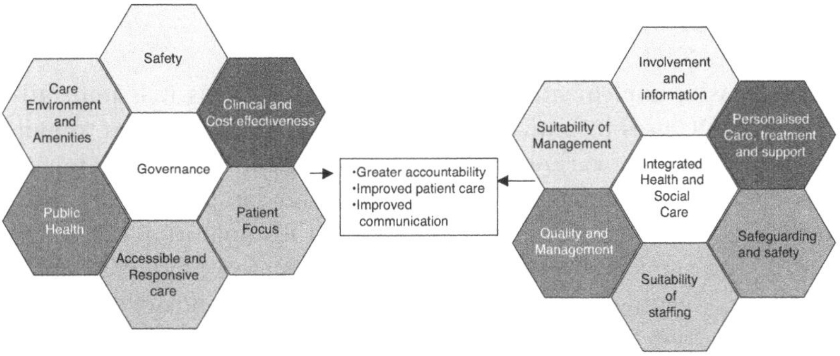

Fig. 2.4 The interdependent relationship of healthcare standards.

of the healthcare standards fit together and that they are interdependent on each other through the use of a whole systems approach to quality improvement.

This approach recognises the need for an integrated approach to health and social care governance, where through the development of interdependent relationships it is more likely to succeed. It can be applied to all health and social organisations as it represents the very core of our business, delivering high-quality patient-focused care locally. We would argue that that this encourages clinical and non-clinical staff to harmonise efforts for the good and benefit of patients in a coordinated and efficient manner.

Both the previous healthcare standards (DH 2004b) and proposed new regulations (CQC 2009a) highlighted in Fig. 2.4 show vast similarities in the way they categories the key elements associated with quality health and social care. These will only be effective through the adoption of a whole systems approach. A whole systems approach reinforces the concept of health and social care governance applicable to any organisation and individual. With the previous standards for better health and new proposed regulations there are some common categories which can be applied and reviewed under the heading of safety and safeguarding, person-centred, quality and management, suitability of staff. The key difference of the proposed new regulations is the inclusion of the terms management which historically has been considered from a governance perspective rather than a management perspective. Both frameworks are associated with competency or performance-related issues at an organisational, department/directorate and team level the same could be used for promoting improvements and quality across health and social care. The key to successful change through the previous healthcare standards and new regulations is associated with harmonising (or integration) of the clinical and non-clinical aspects of governance as is depicted in the next section.

Criteria for evaluating the standards

For successful implementation of the CQC regulations it is imperative that the CQC uses its authority to encourage all inspectorates to unite. Unification of these various organisational accrediting bodies is imperative. The key disadvantage of organisational standards and accreditation within the health and social care today is in the duplication of time, resources and support needed for individuals, teams and organisations in collecting, collating and providing evidence. Health and social care organisations seem to be pressurised not just in meeting the criteria for one award but several at any one time (McSherry *et al.* 2004).

A critical review of the organisational and accreditation frameworks such as Invests in People (IIP), European Foundation for Quality Management (EFQM), CNST and Charter Mark has already revealed a set of the primary core themes in the publication of the Excellence in Practice Accreditation Scheme (EPAS) (McSherry *et al.* 2003). EPAS provides a robust framework supporting the clinical governance agenda because of its associations with the key components of clinical governance. There are many examples of organisational accreditation schemes but none of them capture the essence of clinical governance or evidence-based practice within a practice development framework. The uniqueness of the EPAS is in collectively addressing the key issues in developing, advancing and evaluating practice, which could easily be transferred and further, developed to incorporate the non-clinical aspects of integrated governance model and the healthcare standards.

The acid test for the CQC regulations and ultimately the CQC itself will be in demonstrating a reduction in the burden of inspection, by the use of intelligent information that ultimately leads to targeted and proportionate inspection and improved patient related outcomes and experience.

Activity 2.2 Feedback: non-clinical services that support the implementation of clinical governance.

- Finance
- Personnel (human resources)
- Estates: building, electrical and mechanical services
- Catering
- Domestic services
- Information technology
- Administration and clerical services
- Medical records
- Library services

Note: This is by no means an exhaustive list and is not placed in any order of priority

Activity 2.3 Feedback.

What do you understand by the term national healthcare standards? Why do you think these have been developed? What aspects of health care do you think these standards should cover?

Whilst the previous Standards for Better Health (DH 2004b) adopted a broad approach to performance management taking into consideration the perspectives of the DH, Healthcare Professionals and more importantly patients and carers providing a clear set of standards that all NHS organisations should be meeting.

The introduction of the Care Quality Commission (CQC) has subsumed the role of the Health Care Commission and as such proposed the introduction of a new regulatory framework for assuring quality in health and social care across public and independent sectors. This new approach attempts to integrate the various health and social care structures and systems within an organisation using a whole systems approach which may improvement quality, enhance patient-related outcomes and experience.

Conclusion

In conclusion, clinical governance is a highly complex and multifaceted concept dependent upon successful adoption of a whole systems approach that integrates the clinical and non-clinical services. The successful integration of these various elements within any health and social care organisation we believe could result in the achievement of 'health and social care governance'. Health and social care governance is about establishing frameworks for sustaining and improving quality, which can only take place when the organisational infrastructures support the overall aims of corporate, clinical and non-clinical aspects of governance.

Garside (1999) reinforces our term 'health and social care governance' by suggesting that clinical governance is 'the opportunity to change systems – to pull together different components and strands from the clinical and managerial worlds to improve things for patients'. The challenge for the health and social is in 'converging' all of the governance components identified' in Fig. 2.4 under a single umbrella which all health and social care professionals can access, understand, implement and evaluate at a level most suited to their roles and responsibilities in the attempt to minimise risks. Convergence has already been recognised by the DH: 'We are committed to achieving a fully integrated approach to governance where clinical and corporate governance sits side by side – clinical governance focusing on continuous improvements in quality and corporate governance focusing on having the necessary systems in place to minimise risk'. (Reeves 2001, p. 1). The Health Service Circular 2001/005

(NHS Executive 2001) provides advice and guidance together with a timetable for this to occur within the NHS by 2005. In 2005 the DH introduced the term integrated governance in 2004 and published guidance on what this means for NHS organisations (DH 2006a, 2006b). In 2009 the establishment of the Care Quality Commission (CQC) is a major change fostering collaborative and partnership working through adopting an integrated approach to regulation and review. Whilst we would argue adopting a truly Integrated health and social care governance approach for quality improvement. We believe the term tends to focus on organisational and managerial aspects of a health and social care organisation at higher levels appearing to have limited relevance and application to staff in their daily work. To develop your understandings about clinical governance the key components will be examined in detail in Chapter 3.

Key points

Corporate governance
Corporate governance in general is about protecting investors' monies and companies' assets from risks. Likewise corporate governance in the NHS is about ensuring that public monies have not been wasted in healthcare delivery.

Clinical governance
Clinical governance is a framework for the continual improvement of patient care by minimising clinical risks and continuing the development of organisations and staff.

Healthcare governance
Healthcare governance is the harmonisation of corporate governance, clinical governance and controls assurance.

Health and social care governance
Health and social care governance is the harmonisation of corporate governance, clinical governance across and between health and social care organisations, teams and individuals.

Suggested reading

Hopkins, B. (2000) National Controls Assurance Conference. *Health Care Risk Report*, 6 (3) 22–24.

NHS Executive (1999) *Health Services Circular 1999/123. Governance in the New NHS: Controls Assurance Statements 1999/2000: Risk Management and Organizational Controls*. DH, London.

RCN (2000) *Clinical Governance: How Nurses Can Get Involved*. Royal College of Nursing, London.
Smith, S. (1998) Model behaviour. *Nursing Management*, 5 (6) 19–24.

Useful websites

Australian Council on Health Care Standards (2004) ACHS News Issue 12, Spring 2004. ACHS.
Care Quality Commission (2009) Care Quality Commission http://www.cqc.org.uk/. Accessed 06 August 2009.
The National Institute for Health and Clinical Excellence (2009) Welcome to the National Institute for Health and Clinical Excellence http://www.nice.org.uk/. Accessed 06August 2009.

References

Braithwaite, J. & Travaglia, J.F. (2008). An overview of clinical governance policies, practices and initiatives. *Australian Health Review*, 32 (1) 10–23.
Care Quality Commission (2009a) About CQC http://www.cqc.org.uk/aboutcqc.cfm. Accessed 06 August 2009.
Care Quality Commission (2009b) *National Minimum Standards CQC*. London http://www.cqc.org.uk/guidanceforprofessionals/socialcare/careproviders/nationalminimumstandards.cfm. Accessed 13 August 2009.
Chua-Eoan, H. (1995) *Cover: Leeson Destroys Barings: Going for Broke*. http://www.time.com/time/magazine/archive/1995/950313/950313.cover.html.
Deighan, M., Cullen, R. and Moore, R. (2004) The development of integrated governance. Debate No.3. The NHS Confederation.
Department of Health (2000a) *The NHS Plan: A Plan for Investment, A Plan for Reform*. DH, London.
Department of Health (2000b) *National Service Framework Coronary Heart Disease Modern Standards and Service Models*. DH, London.
Department of Health (2002) *Independent Health Care, National Minimum Standards, Regulations*. DH, London. http://www.dh.gov.uk/en/ Publicationsandstatistics/Publications/PublicationsPolicyAndGuidance/DH_4085259. Accessed 13 August 2009.
Department of Health (2003) *Building on the Best: Choice, Responsiveness and Equity in the NHS*. DH, London.
Department of Health (2009) *NHS Foundation Trusts*. http://www.dh.gov.uk/en/Healthcare/Secondarycare/NHSfoundationtrust/DH_072543. Accessed 06 August 2009.
Department of Health (2004a) http://www.dh.gov.uk/PublicationsAndStatistics/Publications/PublicationsPolicyAndGuidance/PublicationsPolicyAndGuidanceArticle/fs/en?CONTENT_ID=4096679&chk=UCEB%2B1.
Department of Health (2004b) *Standards for Better Health: Healthcare Standards for Services under the NHS – A Consultation Document*. DH, London.

Department of Health (2006a). *Intergrated Governance Handbook: A Handbook for Executives and Non-executive in Healthcare Organisations*. DH, London.
Department of Health (1994) *Corporate Governance in the NHS, Code of Conduct, Code of Accountability*. The Stationery Office, London.
Department of Health (1997) *The New NHS Modern and Dependable*. The Stationery Office, London.
Department of Health (1998) *A First Class Service: Quality in the new NHS*. The Stationery Office, London.
Donaldson, L.J. (1998) Clinical governance: quality improvement as a duty, not a choice. *Healthcare Quality*, 4 (3) 7–9.
Emslie, S. (2001) Controls assurance in the National Health Service in England – the final piece of the corporate governance jigsaw. *Corporate Governance*, 12 March. Abg Professional Information, London.
Garside, P. (1999) Book review. *Clinical Governance: Making it Happen* (eds M. Lugon & J. Secker-Walker). RSM Press, London. *BMJ*, 318, 881.
Healthcare Commission (2009) *Mid Staffordshire NHS Foundation Trust; A Review of Lessons Learnt for Commissioners and Performance Managers Following the Healthcare Commission Investigation*. HCC, London.
Hopkins, B. (2000) National Controls Assurance Conference. *Health Care Risk Report*, 6 (3) 22–24.
McNeil, J. (1998) Clinical governance: the whys, whats, and hows for theatre practitioners. *British Journal of Theatre Nursing*, 9 (5) 208–216.
McSherry, R. & Haddock, J. (1999) Evidence based health care: its place within clinical governance. *British Journal of Nursing*, 8 (2) 113–117.
McSherry, R. & McSherry, W. (2001) Putting research into practice. *Nursing Times*, 97 (23) 36–37.
McSherry R. & Pearce P (2002) *Clinical Governance A Guide to Implementation for Healthcare Professionals*. Blackwell Science Publications: Oxford.
McSherry, R. & Pearce, P. K. (2000) Interpreting the new controls guidelines. *Health Care Risk Report*, 6 (3) 19–21.
MONITOR (2009) *Independent Regulator of NHS Foundation Trusts*. http://www.monitor-nhsft.gov.uk/home. Accessed 06 August 2009.
NHS Choices (2009) *Your Health, Your Choices*. http://www.nhs.uk/nhsengland/NSF/pages/Nationalserviceframeworks.aspx. Accessed 6 August 2009.
NHS Executive (1999) *Health Service Circular 1999/123 Governance in the New NHS: Controls Assurance Statements 1999/2000: Risk Management and Organizational Controls*. DH, London.
NHS Executive (2001) *Health Service Circular 2001/005. Controls Assurance Statements 2000/2001 and Establishment of The Controls Assurance Support Unit*. DH, London.
Pearce, P.K (2004), Controls assurance: benefit or burden? *Governance Matters*, 7 August/September, 5–6.
RCN (2000) *Clinical Governance: How Nurses Can Get Involved*. Royal College of Nursing, London.
Reeves, C. (2001) *Letter: Governance in the NHS*. NHS Executive, Leeds.
Royal College of General Practitioners (2005) Cited in McSherry R., Pearce P. (2007) eds. *Clinical Governance: A Guide to Implementation for Healthcare Professionals*. Blackwell Publishing: Oxford.

Royal College of Nursing (1998) *Clinical Governance: An RCN Resource Guide*. RCN, London.

Royal Pharmaceutical Society of Great Britain (2005) Cited in McSherry R., Pearce P. (2007) eds. *Clinical Governance: A Guide to Implementation for Healthcare Professionals*. Blackwell Publishing: Oxford.

Scally, G. & Donaldson, L.J. (1998), Clinical governance and the drive for quality improvement in the new NHS in England. *BMJ*, 317, 61–65.

Schroeder, P.S. & Maibusch, R.M. (1984). *Nursing Quality Assurance: A Unit Based Approach*. Aspen Publication, Rochville, MD.

Sealey, C. (1999) Clinical governance: an information guide for occupational therapists. *British Journal of Occupational Therapy*, 62 (6).

Smith, R. (1998a) All changed, changed utterly: British Medicine will be transformed by the Bristol Case. *BMJ* 316, 1917–1918.

Vanu Som C (2004) Clinical governance: A fresh look at its definition. *Clinical Governance: An International Journal*. 9 (2) 87–90.

Chapter 3

A Guide to Clinical Governance

Rob McSherry and Paddy Pearce

Introduction

The previous chapters looked at the contributing factors that led to the introduction of clinical governance, and what clinical governance is. This chapter builds on the previous chapter by exploring and explaining in detail the key components of clinical governance by the application and modification of McSherry and Haddock's (1999) framework and by referring to the government's NHS Executive circulars on clinical governance and its associated components.

The key components of clinical governance

As outlined in Chapter 2, clinical governance has several themes associated with its definition: quality improvements and maintenance, professional accountability, creating and maintaining a safe environment for patients and staff along with establishing an honest and open culture that encourages and responds to staff and public opinion – key themes for all healthcare organisations and individuals to develop in pursuit of clinical excellence.

The issue facing many healthcare organisations and individual health professionals is not in distinguishing the key themes associated with clinical governance, because we all want to practise in a clinical environment that proactively develops its staff and services in order to enhance the standards and quality of care, treatments or interventions. The concerns expressed by many healthcare professionals focus on answering the questions of implementing clinical governance for organisations and individuals as highlighted in Box 3.1.

Clinical Governance, third edition. By Rob McSherry and Paddy Pearce.

Box 3.1 Questions associated with describing the key components of clinical governance.

What are the key components of clinical governance?
Is clinical governance only an organisational concern?
How do you implement a system of clinical governance?
Can a clinical governance framework be developed for individual healthcare professionals to use in pursuit of clinical excellence?

Box 3.1 is not an exhaustive list of questions raised by healthcare professionals in highlighting the practicalities of developing and implementing a system of clinical governance. Box 3.1 demonstrates staff's concerns and confusions over what clinical governance has to offer at an organisational, team and individual level in improving the quality and standards of care. Essentially clinical governance is the term used to focus individual and organisational attentions back to quality: 'So that quality is at the core, both of their responsibilities as organisations and of each of their staff as individual professionals' (DH 1997a, p. 47). The government's quote on clinical governance clearly responds to the questions raised in Box 3.1 by suggesting that both individual healthcare professionals and their organisations are to work within the framework of clinical governance.

Activity 3.1 Key components of clinical governance.

In Chapter 2 we identified how clinical governance is about promoting, maintaining and evaluating best practices. To achieve clinical excellence at an individual and organisational level, what systems or infrastructures do you feel should be in place to achieve this goal?

Write down your responses on a sheet of paper and then read on and compare your findings with those at the end of the chapter.

Before outlining the key components of clinical governance it is essential to describe the relationship between the healthcare organisation and the achievement of quality care.

Healthcare organisations and the achievement of quality care

Clinical excellence will flourish in an organisation that proactively responds to incidents, complaints or suggestions by the public or staff regarding their experience of providing or receiving clinical care,

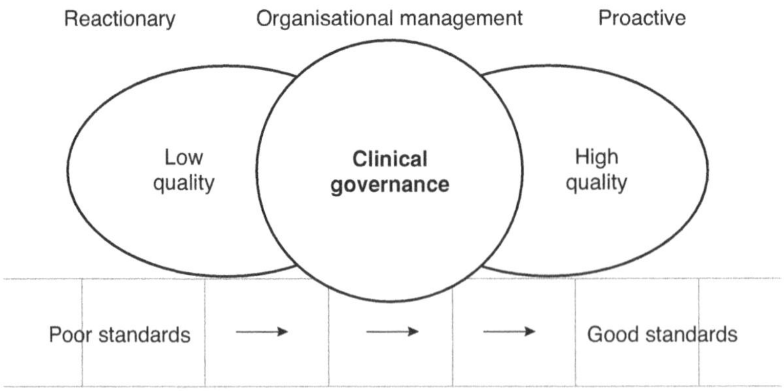

Fig. 3.1 Clinical excellence and its association with organisational management styles.

treatments or interventions from healthcare professionals or service users. Scally and Donaldson (1998) develop the idea of quality dependence and organisational stability/instability in detail by offering an illustration that describes the variations in the quality of health by focusing on low- and high-quality practices. A bell curve is offered with low quality at one end and high quality at the other. Where low or poor quality is experienced, potential problems could exist in the form of untoward incidents and increased complaints; the aim is for healthcare organisations to shift changes in practice from the centre or mean towards the high quality. Whilst the Scally and Donaldson (1998) illustration outlining the variations in the quality of health organisations is a useful way of viewing the standards of quality, it is not without its limitations. For example, how does an organisation establish the mean or best practices for a certain service? How does the organisation or individual know that the standards of practice are of high or low quality?

To address some of the above limitations and to further build on Scally and Donaldson's (1998) work it is important to demonstrate the link between proactive and reactionary organisational management and leadership in achieving clinical excellence, and its association with implementing a clinical governance framework as depicted in Fig. 3.1.

It is clear from Fig. 3.1 that a system of clinical governance will only be achieved where a balance between reactionary and proactive management and leadership exists within the healthcare organisation; this will hopefully result in the continued provision of medium to high quality care. To achieve high quality care it is essential that the right culture and clinical environments and services are created, and this depends on nurturing a proactive approach to management and leadership. That is not to say reactionary management is ineffective, because there may be occasions when this type of approach is advocated. To create an open culture that positively seeks and responds to criticisms and compliments will take time, but it is the preferred style advocated within the clinical governance frameworks and transformational leadership style.

So what are the qualities required by an organisation to become more proactive in nature? Scally and Donaldson (1998) and Donaldson & Muir Gray (1998) indicate that quality improvements are dependent on having an:

> organisation-wide approach to quality improvement with emphasis on preventing adverse outcomes through simplification and improving the process of care. Leadership and commitment from the top of the organisation, team work, consumer focus, and good data are also important (Scally & Donaldson 1998, p. 62).

These are key attributes inferred by having a proactive management approach.

The white paper The New NHS Modern, Dependable (DH 1997a) describes how a quality organisation can be achieved by proactively ensuring that the ten attributes and processes shown in Box 3.2 are present.

Box 3.2 Key attributes associated with promotion of a quality organisation.

- There is an integrated approach to quality improvement throughout the whole organisation.
- Leadership skills are developed in line with professional and clinical needs.
- Infrastructures exist that foster the development of evidence-based practices.
- Innovations are valued and good practices are shared within and without the organisation.
- Clinical risk management systems are in place.
- There is a proactive approach to reporting and dealing with and learning from untoward incidents.
- Complaints are taken seriously and actions taken to prevent any recurrence.
- Ensuring that poor clinical performance is recognised thus preventing potential harm to patients or staff.
- Practice and professional development is aligned and integral to clinical governance frameworks.
- Clinical data is of the best quality and can be used effectively to monitor patient care and clinical outcomes.

Adapted from (DH 1997a)

It is evident from Box 3.2 that the establishment of a proactive organisational culture is dependent on the development of 'effective channels of communication between healthcare professionals' (McSherry & Haddock 1999) and infrastructures such as education, training, research and access to high quality information in supporting staff in their pursuit of clinical excellence. Essentially, 'successful quality improvement demands major cultural change – but that change cannot simply be imposed, as it entails a significant shift in the way that people think and behave' (Walshe *et al.* 2000, p. 1). The question that often remains unanswered in much of the literature reviewed by the authors is, how do you achieve successful culture change(s)?

Figure 3.1 demonstrates how a proactive management and transformational leadership styles are the best way to promote an honest and open culture which can and will only be achieved through strong leadership and commitment to genuine quality improvement. This approach to management, of openly encouraging a shared ownership for the active development, implementation and evaluation of the infrastructures associated with clinical governance, is the key to success. Involvement of staff from all levels within and without the organisation needs to be carefully considered. Without the involvement and cooperation of clinical staff, clinical governance will not make a difference to patient care.

A possible approach for encouraging positive cultural shifts or changes in attitudes is that offered by McSherry & Haddock (1999) in highlighting the key components and structures of evidence-based practice (see Fig. 3.2).

Figure 3.2 describes how the development of the staff's culture is paramount if successful implementation of evidence-based practice in relation to clinical governance is to be achieved. The key components are

Fig. 3.2 Promoting a culture for evidence-based practice within clinical governance. (Reproduced from McSherry & Haddock (1999). Used with permission from MA Healthcare Limited.)

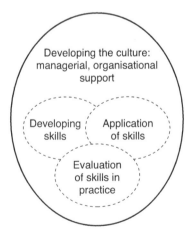

the development, application and evaluation of practices that can be used at organisational and individual levels.

The same approach could be transferred to the development of clinical governance in that the correct organisational culture needs to be established whilst the infrastructures are being developed and implemented. The starting point for healthcare organisations to successfully implement clinical governance is to review the white papers (DH 1997a, 1998) and Department of Health guidance documents, NHS Circular 1999/065 (NHS Executive 1999a), on clinical governance with reference to local internal organisational structures and policies.

It is evident from the information presented thus far, that clinical governance is a highly complex system containing and involving many themes and management and organisational processes in the pursuit of individual and organisational clinical quality. What remains to be described and discussed is how to ensure that clinical governance becomes a reality for all practising healthcare professionals in the NHS and independent sector.

Upon reading the NHS Circular 1999/065 and the literature by Edwards and Packham (1999), McSherry and Haddock (1999) and Donaldson (2000), several key themes emerge that encompass the key elements of clinical governance (Fig. 3.3).

It is evident from Fig. 3.3 that risk management, performance management, quality improvement, information and accountability are central

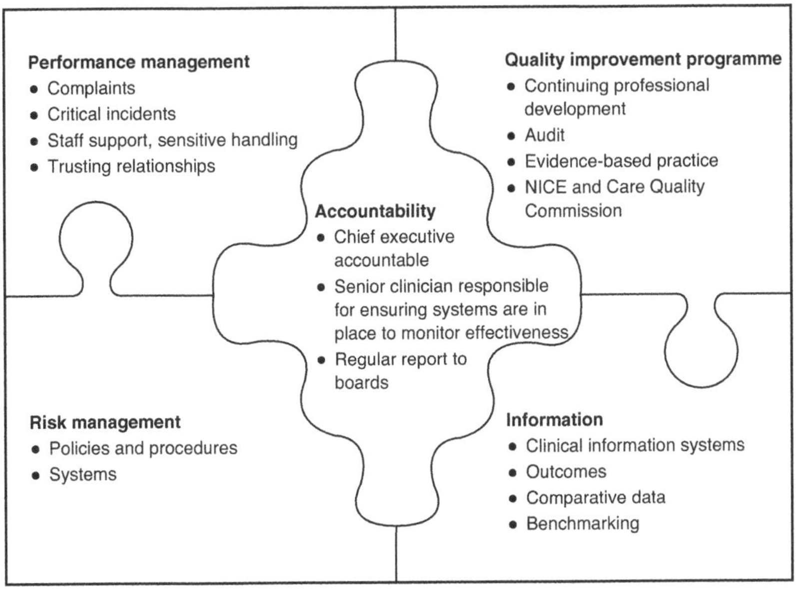

Fig. 3.3 Key components of clinical governance. (Modified from the McSherry & Haddock (1999) template outlining clinical governance. Used with permission from MA Healthcare Limited.)

to the delivery of effective clinical governance. This will now be outlined in more detail.

Risk management

Risk management simply means practising safely: 'It aims to develop good practice and reduce the occurrence of harmful or adverse incidents' (RCN 2000 p. 19). The concept of risk management is about the reduction of clinical and non-clinical risks associated with healthcare. In the past, risk management focused on the financial areas of healthcare.

Over the past decade clinical risk management has become a high priority for the NHS under the auspices of 'Patient Safety'. As a result the National Patient Safety Agency (NPSA) (NPSA 2008) has been established to improve clinical risk management. A fundamental aim of the NPSA in keeping with the principles of clinical governance is to share learning from patients' safety incidents across the NHS and independent sector. It is important to remember when exploring the notion of risk that the following definitions of risk could be applied to either the clinical or non-clinical aspects of healthcare:

- A variation in the outcomes that could occur over a specified period in a given situation (Williams & Heins 1976).
- The possibility of incurring misfortune or loss (Collins 1985)
- The chance or possibility of bad outcome (Wilson & Tingle 1999).
- The probability or likelyhood that harm may occur. Coupled with the consequence of that harm (Mayatt 2004).

Healthcare governance is about the management of 'risk' regardless of its origins within the corporate systems and processes. Some healthcare professionals, teams and organisations tend to view 'risk' in relation to their own position and profession and not in a holistic manner; this may result in only partial reductions and minimisations of a given risk, which may be seen only as a clinical risk. Clinical risk is defined as 'a clinical error to be at variance from intended treatment, care, therapeutic intervention or diagnostic result; there may be an untoward outcome or not' (Wilson & Tingle 1999, p. 71). This notion is evidenced in the following example. Several patients in a specific clinical area develop wound infections resulting in extended lengths of stay, patient discomfort and increased workload and costs for staff working in that organisation. If this situation was identified by a clinician as a professional issue only, they might identify the clinical risk but fail to consider the broader issues surrounding this situation, such as ward cleanliness, adherence to infection control policies and procedures, addressing education and training and overall considerations of resource allocation and finance.

Risk management is mainly 'concerned with harnessing the information and expertise of individuals within the organisation and translating that with their help into positive action which will reduce loss of life, financial loss, loss of staff availability, loss of the availability of buildings or equipment and loss of reputation' (DH 1994). Within the context of healthcare governance the identification and management of risks should be viewed in a holistic way associated with the clinical, environmental and operational aspects of the incident, situation or event.

However, the most important aspect, that of clinical quality, was underdeveloped (DH 2000). This philosophy over the past several years has changed significantly. It would seem that since the lifting of crown immunity in 1995, where central government was responsible for the payment of clinical negligence claims for all NHS organisations, a shift in responsibility to the individual NHS organisations has occurred for the settlement of such claims. This change in policy made NHS organisations seriously consider how their organisation and staff were managing risks. In response to the lifting of crown immunity, NHS Trusts realised the need to address this issue of protecting themselves from the pursuit of clinical negligence claims which would have to be financed from their annual budgets.

The lifting of crown immunity led to the establishment of the Clinical Negligence Scheme for Trusts (CNST) in 1995. These have know been superseded by the National Health Service Litigation Authority (2009) Risk Management Standards. The basic principle of the scheme is similar to a personal, household or car insurance where you pay your premiums and obtain discounts for no-claims. With NHSLA (2009) Risk Management Standards you pay your premiums based on the size of your hospital, its specialties, and on your claims history, and you receive discount for minimising and managing clinical risks. The level of discount is associated with achieving compliance with standards ranging from level one to three. The higher the level of accreditation against the required standards, the greater the discount. Essentially the NHSLA is a pooling scheme for its members where, should a huge negligence claim be made against a Trust, the scheme would pay out the settlement after the Trust had paid its excess (Mayatt 1995).

The NHSLA Risk Management Standards are available for a diverse range of healthcare providers for example, acute hospitals, primary care trusts and independent sector, mental health and learning disability, ambulance and maternity services. The Risk Management standards for all are centred around five generic standards as follows:

Standard 1 – *Governance*: requires evidence of a strategic and systematic approach to risk management and the development, implementing of associated policies/procedures along with evaluation frameworks to establish impact on practice. The standard also covers the importance of developing, maintaining, interrogating and producing information/data from risk registers. Furthermore a robust clinical records management framework and professional registration and education programme/training of the workforce is essential.

Standard 2 – *Competent and capable workforce:* requires a robust and systematic approach to developing, implementing and evaluating the impact of corporate and local induction programmes. The establish of sound systems and processes for the supervision of staff, ensuring staff and patients safety needs, preventing and managing healthcare acquired infection and safe moving and handling. A training needs analysis of the workforce and a framework for responding to external reviews, complaints, incidents and accolades is imperative.

Standard 3 – *Safe environment:* Highlights the importance of developing systems and processes for safeguarding children and adults, the establishment of sound human resources evidence-based policies particularly akin to sickness and absence management, violence and aggression, stress, harassment and bullying. Furthermore environmental and health and safety policies associated with slip, trips, fails, inoculation injury and moving and handling are essential requirements.

Standard 4 – *Clinical care:* is associated with developing, implementing and evaluating communications/information structures, protecting sensitive data, medicines management, dealing with consent, maintaining sound standards for record and record keeping and in ensuring safe transfer and discharge of patients, the management and prevention of infection and ensuring effective opertaionalisation of resuscitation policies, procedures and practices.

Standard 5 – *Learning from experience:* encourages the proactive development of reviewing and learning from incidents, concerns, complaints and claims through the having robust systems and processes for reviewing, investigating and sharing lessons learnt by adopting sound governance principles of honesty, openness and transparency through engaging with best evidence/practices.

The NHSLA Risk Management standards offers a framework to minimise and manage clinical risks in the pursuit of clinical excellence. Initially CNST was intended to reduce financial risks: 'a large settlement or a series of sizable settlements could significantly impinge upon the overall financial position of a Trust' (Mayatt 1995, p. 2). Today CNST or the NHSLA remains a voluntary organisation designed to support the clinical risk aspect of clinical governance. NHSLA Risk management scheme offers a framework for the management of clinical risk, although there continues to be room for ongoing development and improving the clinical risk infrastructures as alluded to by the Chief Medical Officer (DH 2000). An example of improved clinical risk infrastructures could be the establishment of a national incident reporting system to detect potential clinical risks for all NHS organisations at an early stage. The NPSA are currently developing such a scheme. This approach to the management of risks was highlighted in An Organisation with a Memory (DH 2000) and how it will be actioned via Building a Safer NHS for Patients. Implementing an Organisation with a Memory (DH 2001).

It is important to mention here that whilst the CNST standards and NHSLA Risk management Standards have done much to advance risk management and reduce clinical risks, there is a need for a holistic management of 'risk'. The Care Quality Commission (CQC) is currently focusing on developing such an approach to risk management through registration and review processes commencing in January 2010.

Managing performance

The DH (1997a) reforms of the NHS provided a performance assessment framework that supports the drive for higher quality standards by ensuring that performance assessment is focused on the delivery of effective, appropriate and timely health services which meet local needs (DH 1997a, p. 63).

Within the clinical governance framework the management of weak performance of either devices or personnel is imperative in reducing clinical failures. As highlighted earlier in this chapter, management and leadership styles play an important part in how people perform. In addition to having a proactive management style and transformation leadership together with an honest and open culture which encourages staff and the public to express ideas or concerns, how can an organisation detect, promote and deal with good or weak performance?

It is acknowledged within the literature (DH 2000; RCN 2000) that the delivery of health care involves many complex systems and processes involving a diverse range and set of individuals to provide the best service to the public. With this in mind it is easier to apportion blame to individuals rather than the systems when things go wrong. This is because for many organisations reviewing systems is challenging, time consuming and costly, and for some organisations it is about establishing where to start. The easy option is to blame the individual when things go wrong, but this reactionary approach is not beneficial to preventing recurrence of the situation. What is needed is a review of the systems and processes associated with the incident, and to be honest and open with the findings. This type of approach associated with reviewing and learning from incidents, events or failures is encouraged by the NPSA who advocate the use of 'Root Cause Analysis Techniques'.

> A 'Root Cause Analysis (RCA) investigations are a well recognised way of doing this, offering a framework for reviewing patient safety incidents (and claims and complaints). Investigations can identify what, how, and why patient safety incidents have happened. Analysis can then be used to identify areas for change, develop recommendations and look for new solutions. Ultimately, they should help stop incidents from happening again'. (NPSA 2008, p. 1).

This proactive approach to dealing with incidents, complaints, concerns and claims involving individuals, teams or systems and processes requires a major cultural shift, as eloquently described by the Royal College of Nursing:

> A culture that encourages open discussion and reflection on practice allows staff to learn from their experiences. This includes both celebrating what is done well and learning from what is done less well. However, if an organisation is going to encourage clinicians to report incidents and learn from mistakes, it must develop a blame free culture, rather than one that revolves around disciplinary procedures. (RCN 2000, p. 8)

It is evident from the RCN's definition that performance management in healthcare services needs to be reorganised to deal with good and poor performances, as this has not been the case in the past. Achieving this goal is about developing simple but effective systems and processes that capture performances of individuals, teams, organisations and devices which work well and not so well. The overall aim of this type of performance management is to establish, share and learn from the experiences of others in promoting excellence in practice.

Activity 3.2 Performance management.

Write down what you think influences the performance of an individual, team or organisation, along with the systems and processes that should be developed in an organisation to assist in dealing with good or weak performance.

Compare your responses with those in the Feedback box at the end of the chapter.

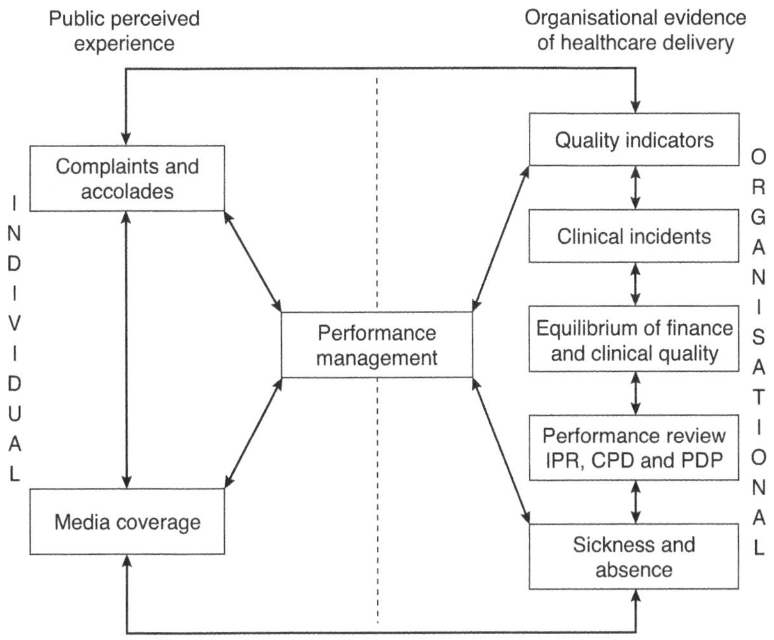

Fig. 3.4 Framework for performance management.

We believe two main factors influence performance management in the NHS: the perceived experiences of the public and the organisation's philosophical approach to performance. Figure 3.4 provides a framework outlining the various components associated with performance management, of which more is explained below.

Figure 3.4 shows how performance management is about dealing with good and not so good performance. It is clear that the public's view is based upon individuals' experience of, or the media coverage of, the services or a combination of both. Often 'all that is good in healthcare is regarded by the public as being attributable to doctors and nurses, while all that is bad is the fault of managers and their political masters' (Baker 1998, p. 137). The quote by Baker is plausible and in some cases may be true, but for performance management to operate effectively within the context of clinical governance frameworks, this conception needs to be challenged. Baker's quote seems to suggest that the public and perhaps many health service staff fail to understand that performance depends on uniting the non-clinical infrastructures with the clinical, along with the processes and systems associated with each. Weak performance can often be the result of systems and process failure rather than individuals. Systems are only as good as the design; if this is ineffective then so is the information or care given as a result. To develop good performance management systems within the context of clinical governance, Acute Trusts, Foundation Trust, Primary Care Trusts or Strategic Health Authority boards need to embrace a philosophy that proactively encourages the concept of performance management. In a simple way they need to be able to answer three questions: What are we doing? How well are we doing it? How do we know we are performing well? These can only be answered by having the appropriate systems and processes in place to collect and disseminate information associated with good and not so good performance related to the clinical and non-clinical aspects of healthcare service.

Figure 3.4 shows that there are several systems and processes that need to be in place to provide information on performance. Performance needs to be considered in line with a whole systems approach, where clinical performance and non-clinical performance are seen as equal. In the past the NHS has tended to focus on financial performance and activity, i.e. the number of patient treatments and length of waiting lists. This information is important and needs to be collected; however, it does not provide managers or the public with any information about the quality of care and services provided or indeed how individuals or systems are performing. A range of quality indicators need to be developed that provide information and evidence either on individual, team or organisational performance. These systems and associated processes need to capture activity from a variety of sources, i.e. organisational, team and individual performance such as pressure sore prevalence and hospital-acquired infections. If we apply these examples to Fig. 3.4 it is evident how systems such as clinical incident reporting, incidents, complaints and accolades monitoring, financial and quality reporting, performance reviews and the recording of sickness and absence, can demonstrate the overall performance of individuals, teams and the organisation. This is because each part of the performance management system includes reviewing and acting on the information given in demonstrating good or not so good practice, which can be highlighted through pooling information gathered from several systems and processes such as the following.

Clinical incident reporting

Clinical incident reporting is required for staff and patients in highlighting any areas where an individual or organisation fails to deliver the appropriate standard of care. Incident reporting offers a framework for the detection of untoward incidents and near misses, which enables action to be taken, lessons to be learnt, practices to be reviewed and information to be shared to prevent any recurrence.

Individual performance review

Individual performance review (IPR) should encourage staff to express and report any concerns about their own individual practices so that continued improvements can be made in the delivery of services and in promoting safe practice. Following an IPR an individual professional or personal development plan should be written and agreed by the parties to enable the individual and department to develop their practices in line with the overall direction of the employing organisation (Martin 2000). With the introduction of Agenda for Change (AfC) (DH 2004a) and the Knowledge and Skills Framework (KSF) (DH 2004b), pay is linked to performance. For a member of staff to progress to the next increment of the scale he/she needs to demonstrates achievement of the competencies agreed in the KSF for the post that he/she holds. This again reaffirms the importance of having an annual IPR and PDP.

Complaints and accolades monitoring

Complaints and accolades monitoring elicits trends and patterns in care delivery, enabling the most appropriate action to be taken or indeed to celebrate areas of good performance.

Sickness and absence monitoring

Sickness and absence monitoring enables either the individual, teams or organisation to evaluate the well-being of personnel and can be used to help explain areas of weak performance, e.g. rising numbers of clinical complaints, incidents, concerns and claims in a clinical or non-clinical area because of staff shortages due to sickness and absence.

The DH and the NHS is beginning to realise the importance of investing in staff and in creating a sound working environment and good working. The work of West & Borrill *et al.* (2000a and 2000b) showed a relationship between staff morale, job satisfaction and mortality. Perhaps this work influenced the development of the Improving Working Lives (IWL) initiative introduced by the DH (DH 2000). Taking West & Borrill *et al.* (2000a and 2000b) and the DH (2000b) work into account it would appear that organisations with higher levels of staff satisfaction and morale have better patient outcomes than NHS organisations with lower levels of staff satisfaction and morale.

In summary, performance management is about the integration and utilisation of data and information obtained from services often viewed with negative connotations, such as clinical incident reporting, complaints and clinical audit. However, these systems and processes should be viewed positively, because they often demonstrate the existence of quality services and standards of practice. Performance management is about the integration of the various systems and sources of information in highlighting the overall quality status of the organisation (Garland 1998).

Quality improvement

'Clinical governance' is about assuring sustainable continuous quality improvement, which can only be achieved by the determined and conscious efforts of the clinical and non-clinical staff who have the appropriate support of their organisation to deliver best practice. To obtain improvements in quality systems there needs to be in place appropriate support to facilitate individuals and organisations in the pursuit of clinical excellence (NHS Executive 1999a) or excellence in practice as is often referred to today (McSherry & Warr 2008). Continuous quality improvement is the route to clinical excellence or excellence in practice. Clinical excellence or excellence in practice can only be achieved by having efficient and effective systems of communication with staff and patients and where infrastructures are established that proactively seek to develop, maintain and monitor the standards and quality of care provided by the organisation and individuals themselves. The words 'vigilant' and 'surveillance' come to mind in ensuring that the term clinical governance becomes an integral part of all daily practices.

Several DH initiatives such as Quality, Innovation, Productivity and Prevention (QIPP) (National Health Service Institute for Innovation and Improvement 2009 p 1) is designed to create 'an environment in which change and improvement can flourish; it is about leading differently and in a way that fosters a culture of innovation; and it is about providing staff with the tools, techniques and support that will enable them to take ownership of improving quality of care'. Similarly the Patients Related Outcomes Measures (PROMS, DH 2008c) initiatives according to the University of Oxford (2009, p. 1) aims to 'provide a means of gaining an insight into the way patients perceive their health and the impact that treatments or adjustments to lifestyle have on their quality of life. These instruments can be completed by a patient or individual about themselves, or by others on their behalf'. Both QIPP and PROMs illustrate the constant need to improve the quality of care in the pursuit of excellence and in providing evidence of patient involvement and experience in their care which we believe should be firmly embedded and developed as part of the clinical governance agenda.

The introduction of the World Class Commissioning (DH 2008a) describe commissioning as:

> the process of deciding what services or products are needed, acquiring them and ensuring that they meet requirements. In the NHS, commissioners act on behalf of the public, ensuring they have access to the services they need, not only today but also in the future. World class commissioning is a statement of intent, aimed at delivering outstanding performance in the way we commission health and care services.

Taking the DH (2008a) description of commissioning into account it is imperative that both commissioners and providers of health care are aware of the importance of continuous quality improvements as part of the clinical governance agenda. Both commissioners and providers of health care have an equal duty and responsibility to improve health care where information and data obtained by those who use or provide the service should be obtained to enhance the quality and standards of health care.

Figure 3.5 highlights how clinical excellence can be achieved by having an organisation that continually seeks to improve its standards and practices by having integrated systems of clinical risk management, clinical audit, and practices based on sound-evidence-based research which form the basis of staff development.

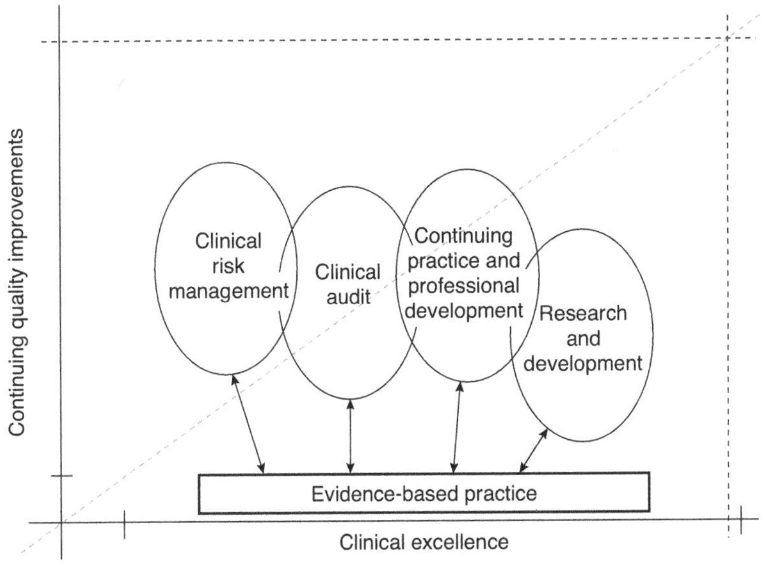

Fig. 3.5 Continuous quality improvement: the route to clinical excellence.

It becomes apparent from Fig. 3.5 that quality improvement is based around the following robust systems and processes:

- Clinical risk management and clinical audit
- Continued practice and professional development
- Implementing continuous professional development within an NHS or independent sector organisation
- Research and development
- Evidence-based health care

Clinical risk management and clinical audit

As outlined previously in this chapter, risk management is about the development of robust systems which assist staff in establishing efficient and effective standards of care against local, national or international standards, in an attempt to minimise and proactively manage risks.

Clinical audit is defined as the systematic and critical review of systems and processes of care, a method that is essential in order to compare performance against evidence-based standards, for example compliance with National Institute for Health and Clinical Excellence (NICE) guidelines. NICE has been responsible for the appraisal and assessment of new and existing technologies and for producing guidelines for the NHS. Clinical audit is the tool to measure compliance of treatment, interventions or care offered to patients, and the resulting effectiveness on patient care. Areas of weak practice or potential risk should be highlighted so that standards or local policies and guidelines can be written to prevent incidents or harm to patients.

Continued practice and professional development

To ensure that an organisation and staff deliver a high quality service they need to have sound knowledge and well developed skills and competencies to perform their roles efficiently and effectively. Lifelong learning and continuing professional development (CPD) should be seen as an ongoing process in ensuring that practices are the most effective and up to date. The term CPD was originally mentioned in the government's white papers (DH 1997a, 1998) where the government set out its long-term goal of modernising the NHS, with the key focus for change centred on quality improvements. In order to achieve this, healthcare organisations must have robust systems and processes to ensure the continued professional development of all their employees.

CPD is defined as:

> A process of lifelong learning for all individuals and teams which meets the needs of patients and delivers the health outcomes and healthcare priorities of the NHS and which enables professionals to expand and fulfil their potential. (DH 1998, p. 42)

CPD should be seen as the beginning of a process of developing a culture of lifelong learning for all staff. To develop a robust system and process for the delivery of CPD local ownership is essential. We do recognise that this is a long-term objective, will take several years to achieve and requires the backing from the chairs and chief executives of healthcare organisations because they have a key role to play in ensuring CPD via collaboration and communication between managers, human resources, nursing and medical education committees, and in ensuring that the educational aspect of CPD meets their organisation's and professional staff's requirements. CPD is for all parts of the NHS; with the increasingly competitive labour market the NHS needs to pay attention to the development of managers and information technology personnel in order to ensure access to current information in supporting the development of their employees and services. To facilitate the development of a system for CPD within a healthcare organisation or team or for individuals, it is imperative to action the points outlined in the Health Service Circular 1999/154 Continuing Professional Development: Quality in The New NHS (NHS Executive 1999b). To illustrate how this can be achieved, the following example is taken from Pearce & McSherry (2000).

Implementing continuing professional development within an NHS organisation

In order to implement HSC 1999/154 within the NHS, individual organisations need to adopt a focused approach to ensure the delivery of high quality care, an approach that could be enhanced by the development of robust CPD. In applying this principle the concept of 'management' by objectives could be introduced. This style of managing CPD enables the Trust to anticipate and highlight important issues relevant to the needs of their healthcare population. Corporate objectives are set prior to the start of the financial year, which are specific to the core elements of the organisation's business plan. From these core objectives, sub-objectives for clinical and general managers are established and linked to the personal development plans (PDP) for their staff. A PDP is linked to the individual's annual performance appraisal where the employee and manager review the year's progress and assess strengths, weaknesses, opportunities and

Phase 1	February/March
Corporate objectives to executive directors	

Phase 2	April
Executive and general clinical managers agree objectives to address corporate objectives	

Phase 3	April
General and clinical managers and heads of department agree objectives of their respective departments	

Phase 4	April
Employees and line managers agree individual objectives and personal development plans in line with the Knowledge and Skills Framework (DH 2004b)	

Fig. 3.6 A model to aid the facilitation of CPD into healthcare organisations.

threats (SWOT analysis), jointly agreeing a personal development plan for the next twelve months with a six-monthly review. This approach enables the Trust to systematically identify the important national, regional and local issues to inform a coherent and coordinated strategy in achieving the objectives. This approach to CPD ensures that the Trust is working collaboratively as a team. Figure 3.6 illustrates a model for the CPD processes.

CPD will be discussed in more detail in Chapter 4, but it is worth noting here that CPD is a key element of the Investors in People Award and which many healthcare organisations and teams aspire to (for more information on this award visit the website http:www.iip.co.uk. CPD also forms a major part of the NHS Improving Working Lives standard (IWL) (DH 2000), which all NHS organisations need to attain. It is evident from the above information that CPD and lifelong learning are integral aspects of the clinical governance framework and can only be achieved by mutual collaboration, respect, openness and honesty between employees and employers about how the individual and the organisation are performing. Successful implementation of clinical governance depends on adequate resourcing and genuine commitment from all parties involved, i.e. from the DH to the individual member of staff.

Research and development (R&D)

Research and development is an integral part of clinical governance. The 'R' (research) aspect is often associated with the generation of new, and testing of existing, knowledge. The 'D' aspect for (development) is often unsupported and undervalued in many healthcare organisations, e.g. within clinical governance, staff are expected to be research aware although little resource is allocated in supporting this need (McSherry *et al.* 2006). One aspect of research and development is concerned with establishing ways of enhancing health by the introduction of research. For more information on R&D view the DH Research and Development website: http://www.dh.gov.uk/en/Researchanddevelopment/DH_476

To promote evidence-based practice a system for accessing, implementing, monitoring, supporting, supervising and disseminating research findings should be established to ensure that clinical practices and patient care are based on the most recent and best available scientific evidence, commonly referred to as evidence-based practice. So what is evidence-based practice? The following sections are based on McSherry and Haddock (1999) with kind permission of Mark Allen Publishers Ltd.

Evidence-based healthcare

Evidence-based practice is 'the process of systematically finding and using contemporaneous research findings as the basis for clinical decision-making' (Long & Harrison 1996) and is an integral part of the clinical governance framework, as illustrated in Figs. 3.2 and 3.5. For the successful implementation of clinical governance for organisations and individuals, it is essential that all systems, processes, infrastructures and health professionals are developed using the principles of evidence-based practice. To facilitate the development of evidence-based practice the following processes need to be applied (Kitson 1997; Cullum *et al.* 1998; Swage 1998; McSherry *et al.* 2001):

- Identify areas in practice from which clear clinical questions can be formulated.
- Identify the best-related evidence from available literature.
- Critically appraise the evidence for validity and clinical usefulness.
- Implement and incorporate relevant findings into practice.
- Subsequently measure performance against expected outcomes or against peers.
- Ensure staff are supported and developed through adequate resourcing of evidence-based practice education and training programmes.

For example, to develop an evidence-based organisational strategy for clinical risk management, in ensuring the systematic delivery of appropriate and safe health care by the organisation and all its employees, healthcare professionals require regular clinical exposure and experience (Cullum *et al.* 1998) This is essential in order for them to become familiar and competent in rationalising the risks and benefits of a particular treatment, intervention or delivery of care, to deal with the patient's unique individual set of circumstances. It should only be allowed to occur following a structured period of education and supervision, and when the individual feels competent to do the procedure without assistance.

The continued clinical exposure, observations and experience of new treatments or interventions should in addition be supported by the relevant research evidence where patient participation is reflected in the final choice of treatment, intervention or application of care. The development of healthcare professionals to equip themselves with the critical appraisal skills required to rationalise the risks and benefits of care, and indeed to critique research evidence, requires organisational leadership and service support, sufficient resources and indeed a change in the culture to enable staff to work in this way. Therefore in order for evidence-based practice to function within the context of clinical governance and to truly exist and operate effectively, the key components and structures illustrated in Fig. 3.2 are required.

Figure 3.2 illustrates that it is essential that efficient and effective channels of communication and information-giving are established to promote a culture that proactively develops infrastructures that nurture professional and practice development in the pursuit of clinical excellence (McCormack *et al.* 2004; McSherry & Warr 2008). This can only be achieved by ensuring that the services provided are staffed with appropriately skilled, knowledgeable and competent practitioners who are then actively supported to further develop, apply and evaluate the care or service provided, with the aim of improving the quality and standards of care and treatment delivered to patients. McCormack *et al.* (2004) argue that evidence-based practice is dependent on the creation of an appropriate environment and culture, which facilitates the development of evidence-based care. This approach makes it is essential for healthcare professionals to know how and where to access and appraise the evidence.

Locating the evidence

The following is a guide to where research evidence may be obtained in supporting clinical practices:

- Libraries, local/national
- Voluntary and support organisations
- Clinical audit departments
- Centres for research and development
- Practice development centres
- Centre for reviews and dissemination (York)
- Professional bodies
- Local universities

- Information technology centres
- Electric computerised databases (CINHAL, MEDLINE)
- The Cochrane Library
- The National Electronic Library for Health (NeLH)
- Expert advice

A fundamental problem facing some healthcare professionals after obtaining the relevant information or research evidence is the process of critical appraisal, i.e. how do you evaluate the information? Is it useful, reliable and relevant? This was highlighted by Swage (1998): 'many nurses (indeed all health professionals) stumble at the first hurdle because they are not confident about understanding research and reviews'.

Evidence-based care and the need for critical appraisal skills

Crombie (1996), Sackett *et al.* (1997) and Swage (1998) suggest that critical appraisal is about considering the relevance of a research question, evaluating the evidence collected to answer the question and assessing the effectiveness of the conclusion and the recommendation of the evidence. In a simple way it is about systematically reviewing and questioning the stages of the research process, i.e. title and abstract, introduction/literature review, methods, results, discussions and recommendations, and asking the following questions (adapted from Crombie 1996):

- Is the research of interest?
- Why was it done?
- How was it performed?
- Who was it done to?
- What did it show?
- What is the possible implication for your practice?
- What next: information only, uninteresting or support practice?

Having had the education and training to critically appraise research, in the hope of practising evidence-based care, why is it that so many healthcare professionals continue to base practice around tradition or rituals despite research evidence showing the contrary? Perhaps this is because of some of the barriers to implementation.

Barriers to implementation of the evidence

An enormous amount of literature continues to flood the academic journals relating to all professional groups, suggesting that the theory-practice gap continues to widen (McSherry 1997; May *et al.* 1998; Glacken 2002). To instigate evidence-based care at a clinical level, perhaps organisations and staff need to become familiar with these barriers and begin to develop realistic strategies to overcome them. Healthcare professionals need to challenge these barriers in the continued attempt to improve their quality and standards of clinical practices in light of rising patient expectations and recent government reforms (Chapter 1).

The barriers that continue to be faced by many are:

- Attitudes towards research
- Lack of confidence, understanding and the skills to critically appraise
- Insufficient time within work commitments
- Lack of support from peers, managers and other health professionals
- Lack of resources
- Resistance to change.

Despite attempts to implement research evidence to support practices, many staff continue to experience difficulty with ensuring that the care and treatment they provide is evaluated effectively. Barriers are explored in more detail in Chapter 6.

Evaluation of the evidence

It is important that, following the implementation of research findings on delivering care and treatments, we continue to evaluate the quality, standard and effectiveness of our intervention with regards to the patients' outcomes or benefits to the service or organisation. There are many ways in addition to peer review that this can be achieved:

- Clinical audit
- Comparing standards against national guidance, e.g. NICE, Scottish Intercollegiate Guidelines Network (SIGN), Royal Colleges Guidelines.
- Using a performance management framework
- Benchmarking: the use of comparative performance, i.e. comparing standards and outcomes against similar organisations. Involvement in National Audits performed by the Royal College of Physicians on Stroke and continence care.
- Improvement reviews and performance conducted by the former Healthcare Commission and the Care Quality Commission.

In summary should efficient and effective systems of continuous professional development, research and development, clinical risk and clinical audit be established, the overall cultural emphasis shifts from a reactive nature, i.e. acting on complaints from an unfortunate incident or on area of poor practice or performance resulting from either an individual or service failure – to a more proactive nature, in trying to avoid the incident from happening in the first place (McSherry & Haddock 1999).

In order to make continuous quality improvement in organisations, teams and individuals, quality information is needed.

Quality information

For healthcare professionals and organisations to deliver quality standards, effective communication and information-giving are essential. Communication is defined as 'the exchange of information for some purposes' (McCabe & Timmins 2006). This broad definition of communication is pertinent when exploring clinical governance because it emphasises the enormous task in hand for all healthcare professionals in tailoring their services to the client group and clinical setting and in exchanging the relevant information with the patient, carers, the public and fellow professionals. Information-giving refers to the 'the knowledge acquired through experience or study' Collins (1985). To provide quality information healthcare professionals need to have the knowledge, understanding and effective communication skills to exchange and receive information with and from their patients, carers and colleagues. The Audit Commission (1992) acknowledged that healthcare organisations and processes are complex, reinforcing the need for effective communication with patients about the clinical and non-clinical aspects of care. The report stated that 'lack of information and problems in communicating with health professionals usually come at the top of patients' concerns' (Audit Commission 1992), an issue that continues to remain current. To address the concerns of patients and indeed the public with regard to poor communication and information-giving, many government initiatives were introduced to improve communications within the NHS (Box 3.3).

Box 3.3 Government initiatives aimed at improving communication and information-giving.

- *The Patient's Charter: Raising the Standards* (DH 1992a)
- *The Citizen's Charter* (DH 1992b)
- *Code of Openness in the NHS* (DH 1997b)
- Data Protection Act 1998
- Health Service Circular 1999/053, *For the Record: Managing Records in NHS Trusts and Health Authorities* (NHS Executive 1999c)
- *Information for Health* (NHS Executive 2000a)
- The Caldicott Report (NHS Executive 2000b)
- *Our Health, Our Care, Our Say* (DH 2006)

When referring to Box 3.3 and reflecting upon these documents it is easy to see the importance the government is placing on communication and information-giving to address the issues around poor communication and the stress and anxiety this causes patients and professionals alike. Effective communications are an integral aspect of clinical governance; furthermore communication within and between the key processes is vital in ensuring quality services. Communication and information-giving can be enhanced by auditing communications processes along with paying attention to the quality of information provided. In the Code of Openness in the NHS (DH 1997b) the principles of good communication and information-giving are provided based around access to information, explanations, reasons for decisions and actions and information about what information is available. We believe that information should be given as outlined in Box 3.4.

Box 3.4 Principles of effective information-giving.

The information must be:

- Accurate: Factually correct.
- Timely: Given at the right stage of the process or intervention required.
- Current: Update to with appropriate evidence.
- Easily accessible: Should be provided in several formats, i.e. computer based, leaflets.
- Clear and concise: Simple and easy to understand or follow.
- Audience specific: To consider ethnicity, disability and be provided in a sensitive manner.
- Relevant: Focused and specific detail.

Note: When producing patient information leaflets or when sending information to patients, the Plain English Society could be contacted or any other relevant organisations such as the Charter Mark.

It is evident from Boxes 3.3 and 3.4 and the previous paragraphs that communication and information are important aspects in ensuring clinical excellence for patients, as well as being essential factors for the successful implementation, monitoring and evaluation of clinical governance systems and processes. To demonstrate the effectiveness of clinical governance arrangements within healthcare organisations, information and effective communication are vital.

Information requirements for effective clinical governance systems

Quality information within the clinical governance framework is essential and information needs to be considered at four levels within the NHS: healthcare organisations, teams, individuals.

Healthcare organisations

As clinical governance is about sustained improvement in the care provided by the health service there is a requirement to demonstrate that this is happening. To do this a vast amount of clinical and non-clinical information is required. The Commission for Health Improvement (CHI) had the responsibility for reviewing the clinical governance arrangements of NHS Trusts, Health Authorities, and Primary Care Trusts (PCTs). Chi originally planned to perform clinical governance reviews (CGR) on a four yearly cycle, i.e. to review clinical governance in all NHS organisations every four years. An important aspect of CHI's CGR is the analysis of information provided by the organisation. CHI was disbanded in 2003 and its role of critically reviewing the performance of NHS organisation transferred to The Commission for Healthcare Audit and Inspection, commonly known today as 'The Healthcare Commission' (HC). During its lifespan CHI carried out Clinical Governance Reviews in the majority of NHS organisations in England along with undertaking a number of investigations (CHI 2004). These can be broadly summarised into service failures and inappropriate professional behaviours (CHI 2004). Since the introduction of the HC two principal aims seem to emerge. To reduce the burden of inspection upon the NHS and to make review and inspection more target and proportionate. They intended to do this by the use of intelligent information, i.e. using performance information that currently exists informed by reviews and inspections performed by other agencies and regulators such as the NHSLA, AC and the Health and Safety Executive (HSE) to name but a few. In 2008 the Healthcare Commission has been replaced by the Care Quality Commission (CQC) (CQC 2008) who hope to enhance the role by taking a holistic view regarding the assurance and quality of health and social care.

To meet the challenges posed by the introduction of clinical governance we suggest that clinical governance leads in Trusts read and reflect upon this CQC documents and use it as a basis for the development of the Trust's information strategies and in supporting their clinical governance frameworks. Further information is available at: http://www.cqc.org.uk/

Information for clinical teams

To facilitate clinical governance at the clinical team level, all clinical teams need information on how well they are performing. The types of data and information required to support this process can be categorised into those associated with quantitative (numerical/statistical information) and qualitative (patient and staffing experience) or a combination of both, as with complaints reporting you need numbers and trends to detect patterns, and also the qualitative information about individual complaints or letter of commendation. Likewise this could apply to infection control issues. Examples of quantitative and qualitative information are:

- *Activity*: Numbers of patients treated, e.g. finished consultant episodes (FCEs), average length of stay (LOS), etc.
- *Quality:* Quality indicators (QI), incidence of infections, complaints, pressure sore prevalence rates
- *Outcome measures:* Data pertaining to improved quality of life for the patient for mobility, pain, which is obtained from the use of validated measurement tools, e.g. SF36, Hospital Anxiety Depression Scale, Barthel Index, etc.
- *Readmissions*: These could be unplanned, i.e. patients returning to ITU, CCU or discharged patients being re-admitted soon after discharge.
- *Clinical incidents*: Any untoward incident that can potentially affect the patient's outcome, e.g. drug errors, breakdowns in communication affecting patient care, inappropriate care, etc.
- Health and safety incidents: e.g. falls, accidents at work, factors affecting moving and handling for staff and patients, etc.
- *Benchmarking:* Comparative information between similar clinical and non-clinical teams regarding team performance in standards and quality of care, e.g. stroke audit, UK trauma and audit network, Standards for Better Health (DH 2004a), Care Quality Commission (CQC 2008)
- *Accreditation:* Verification of the standards and quality of care/interventions against set standards, e.g. Kings Fund accreditation website http://www.kingsfund.org.uk/ Charter Marks website http://www.barony.co.uk/chartermark.htm#

Individuals (healthcare professionals and patients)

Healthcare professionals

The clinical governance framework provides infrastructures that facilitate the continued professional development of individuals, which should be aligned to contracts of employment, the KSF (DH 2004b), Human Resources policies and procedures that are all linked to the concept of lifelong learning. To support the integration of lifelong learning and the continued professional development of staff, supporting structures, such as the following, need to be in place to encourage this process:

- Organisational objectives
- Performance appraisal aligned to KSF (as outlined previously in this chapter)
- Personal development plans (PDPs)

- Principles of honesty and openness
- Access to education and training
- Access to adequate and appropriate resources
- Management support, e.g. whistle blowing policy and procedures.
- Proactive rather than reactive approaches to untoward incidents or complaints.
- The development of a learning organisation and culture.

Patients

The public needs to be assured that they will not only receive the best quality service and care but will be active partners directly involved with this provision. Where required, special groups or individuals will be involved in service evaluations and developments such as developing service for individuals with disability, e.g. deafness, learning disabilities, etc... Patients should be actively encouraged to participate in health service development, planning, implementation, delivery and evaluation. The accessing of Local Involvement Networks (LINKS) (DH 2008b) which embraces a joined up approach to patient, client, carer and or user involvement within health and social care and local government should be instrumental in facilitating and monitoring this process. Today patients need to be regarded as equal partners in the development, planning, implementation, delivery and evaluation of services (DH 2008b).

In summary, quality information is essential to achieve effective infrastructures for the implementation, monitoring and evaluation of the systems and processes associated with clinical governance. 'Good communication (information-giving and receiving) flow is fundamental to clinical governance and accountability' (O'Neill 2000, p. 816). Accountability is our final piece of the jigsaw in Fig. 3.3, which will now be explored in more detail in relation to clinical governance.

Accountability

Figure 3.3 illustrates how clinical governance is everybody's business, with all clinical and non-clinical staff responsible for ensuring that they are actively involved with managing and minimising clinical risks. This can only be accomplished if they have the necessary knowledge, understanding and skills to perform their roles efficiently and effectively. Continuous quality improvement is at the heart of all practices, which are regularly monitored with a view to improved performance based on a foundation of efficient and effective channels of communication and information-giving. In essence accountability can be defined as 'the requirement that each nurse (healthcare professional) is answerable and responsible for the outcome of his or her professional actions' (Pennels 1997).

Accountability within the context of clinical governance could be viewed on three levels: organisation, team and individual, all having the responsibility for implementing, monitoring and evaluating the key components of clinical governance within their role. For example, the Trust board's chief executive is accountable to parliament in ensuring compliance of best clinical practice, which is founded on the principles of clinical governance. This can only be achieved and demonstrated by having robust systems of communication, risk management, performance management, quality improvement programmes and effective information systems. Likewise a team (ward/unit/department/GP/Genaral Dental Practitioner surgeries) needs to have similar systems to demonstrate the delivery of best practice.

It is clear from Fig. 3.3 that if you base your practice on these key principles your accountability to the public, employer, patients and profession can only be enhanced along with the standard and quality of care offered. In light of the recent healthcare reforms and media interest in health care (Chapter 1), it is essential that you become familiar with what accountability truly means. 'Accountability is like pregnancy – you cannot be slightly pregnant and you cannot be slightly accountable' (Glover 1999). To be truly accountable and fit for practice we would suggest that you address the following questions:

- What are the contributing factors for change in individual and professional practice?
- What might be the consequences of not changing or developing professional practice?
- How can you ensure that your practice is evidence-based?
- How do you know that your practice is efficient and effective

You will then be equipped with the knowledge, understanding and skills to support your professional accountability. If you familiarise yourself with the issues contained within this chapter and adopt the principles of lifelong learning to address any subsequent gaps in your own knowledge and skills, you will be demonstrating your ability to justify clinical judgements relating to accountability, legal and professional issues and subsequent advances in your practice.

Conclusion

This chapter has outlined in detail the key components of clinical governance and their relationship to organisations, teams and individuals in the pursuit of clinical excellence. The challenges for many healthcare professionals are not in describing or explaining what clinical governance is, but in applying and working with this concept in their daily practice(s). Chapter 4 provides practical advice and guidance on how clinical governance could be implemented to support the organisation, teams and individuals. We would suggest that clinical governance will only become truly effective where the public are an integral part of the process. That is when the patients, carers and service users inform healthcare professional and their employing organisations of when things go well or not so well. Service improvement, development and innovation can no longer be left in the hands of healthcare professionals alone.

Activity 3.1 Feedback: Key components of clinical governance.

It is evident from the contents of this chapter that clinical governance is dependent on having an organisational culture that is open, honest and transparent in the way it deals with untoward incidents, complaints and accolades derived from internal or external sources, i.e. staff or public. To foster this type of culture a managerial style that proactively encourages staff development and continuous learning is fundamental if an organisation aims to achieve continuous quality improvements. Quality improvements are the overriding aim of clinical governance, which is dependent on having the correct systems and processes in place to assure quality for the organisation, teams and individuals. The following systems and processes need to operate efficiently, effectively and harmoniously if clinical governance is to be successful at all these levels of a healthcare organisation:

- Risk management
- Performance management
- Quality improvement programmes
- Information
- Accountability.

Activity 3.2 Feedback: performance management.

It is evident from the section on performance management that several factors may have a positive or negative impact on an individual's, team's or organisation's performance, such as the following:

- Management
- Culture
- Environment
- Effective communication.

Issues surrounding either the individual's, team's or organisation's 'performance' are associated with the above factors, which are primarily communicated via two sources: the public's perceived experiences of a healthcare provision and the organisational evidence such as untoward incidents, clinical complaints and quality outcomes

Key points

- Clinical governance is about promoting and achieving continuous improvement within healthcare organisations and professional practice
- Clinical excellence is dependent on having a proactive management and leadership style and honest and open culture
- Innovations and good practices are shared and lessons learnt from not so good practices
- Clinical governance is dependent on the unification, integration and harmonisation of six key systems and processes contained within a healthcare organisation:
  - Risk management
  - Performance management
  - Quality improvement
  - Information
  - Accountability
  - Communication.
- Lifelong learning, continuous professional development and the integration of evidence into practice through robust research and development infrastructures, are of paramount importance in achieving quality improvements within the clinical governance frameworks.
- Patients, carers and service users should be viewed as an integral and equal partner of service development, planning, implementation, delivery and evaluation

Suggested reading

Baker, M. (1998) *Making Sense of the NHS White Papers*, 2nd edn. Radcliffe Medical Press, Oxford.

Borrill, C.A., West, M. (2000a), *How Good is Your Team? A Guide for Team Members*, Aston Centre of Health Service Organisation Research (ACHSOR), University of Aston, Birmingham.

Borrill, C.A., West, M. (2000b), *Developing Team-working in Health Care: A Guide for Managers*, Aston Centre of Health Service Organisation Research (ACHSOR), University of Aston, Birmingham.

Department of Health (2000) An organization with a memory; report of an expert group on learning from adverse incidents in the NHS chaired by the Chief Medical Officer. DH, London.

Muir Gray, J.A. (1997) *Evidence-Based Healthcare: How to Make Health Policy and Management Decisions.* Churchill Livingstone, London.

National Health Service Institute for Innovation and Improvement (2009) Guest Editorial IN THE DRIVER'S SEAT: Using service improvement tools to drive up quality, drive out inefficiencies and drive down costs. http://www.institute.nhs.uk/nhs_alert/guest_editorials/July_2009_Guest_Editorial.html. Accessed 18 September 2009.
National Health Service Litigation Authority (2009) Risk Management. http://www.nhsla.com/RiskManagement/. Accessed 18 September 2009.
National Patients Safety Agency (2008) National patient safety agency. http://www.npsa.nhs.uk/. Accessed 18 September 2009.
National Patients Safety Agency (2008) Root Cause Analysis. http://www.npsa.nhs.uk/nrls/improvingpatientsafety/patient-safety-tools-and-guidance/rootcauseanalysis/. Accessed 18 September 2009.
NHS Executive (1999a) *Health Service Circular 1999/065 Clinical Governance: Quality in the New NHS*. DH, London.
NHS Executive (1999b) *Health Service Circular 1999/154 Continuing Professional Development: Quality in the New NHS*. DH, London.
O'Neill, S. (2000) Clinical governance in action part 4: communication. *Professional Nurse*, 16 (1) 816–817.
Oxford University (2009) Patient-Reported Outcome Measures (PROMs) http://phi.uhce.ox.ac.uk/home.php. Accessed 18 September 2009.
Pearce, P. & McSherry, R. (2000) Development: making it happen. *Health Care Risk Report*, 6 (10) 15–17.
RCN (2000) *Clinical Governance: How Nurses can get Involved*. Royal College of Nursing, London.
Sealey, C. (1999) Clinical governance; An information guide for occupational therapists. *British Journal of Occupational Therapy*, 62 (6) 263–268.
Squire, S. & Cullen, R. (2001) Clinical governance in action part 7: effective learning. *Professional Nurse*, 16 (4) 1014–1015.
Wilson, J. & Tingle, J. (eds) (1999) *Clinical Risk Modification: A Route to Clinical Governance*. Butterworth Heinemann, Oxford.

References

Audit Commission (1992) *What Seems to be The Matter? Communication between Hospitals and Patients*. Audit Commission, London.
Baker, M. (1998) *Making Sense of the NHS White Papers*, 2nd edn. Radcliffe Medical Press, Oxford.
Care NHS Executive (1999a) *Health Service Circular 1999/065 Clinical Governance: Quality in the New NHS*. DH, London.
Care Quality Commission (2008) *Care Quality Commission* http://www.cqc.org.uk/. Accessed 18 September 2009.
Collins, W. (1985) *The New Collins Concise Dictionary*. Guild Publishing Company, London.
Commission for Health Improvement Investigations (2004) *Lessons From CHIA Investigations 2000–2003*. MHSO, London.

Crombie, I.K. (1996) *The Pocket Guide to Critical Appraisal.* BMJ Publishing Group, London.
Cullum, N., DiCenso, A. & Ciliska, D. (1998) Implementing evidence based nursing; Some misconceptions. *Evidence Based Medicine*, 1 (2) 38–40.
Department of Health (1992a) *The Patient's Charter; Raising the Standards.* The Stationery Office, London.
Department of Health (1992b) *The Citizen's Charter.* The Stationery Office, London.
Department of Health (1994) *Corporate Governance in the NHS, Code of Conduct, Code of Accountability.* The Stationery Office, London.
Department of Health (1997a) *The New NHS Modern, Dependable.* Department of Health, London.
Department of Health (1997b) *Code of Openness in the NHS.* The Stationery Office, London.
Department of Health (1998) *Quality in the New NHS.* Department of Health, London.
Department of Health (2000) *An Organisation With a Memory; Report of an Expert Group on Learning from Adverse Incidents in the NHS Chaired by the Chief Medical Officer.* Department of Health, London.
Department of Health (2001) *Building a Safer NHS for Patients: Implementing an Organisation with a Memory.* Department of Health, London.
DH (2004a) *Agenda for Change: What will it Mean for You? A Guide for Staff.* DH, London.
DH (2004b) *The Knowledge and Skills Framework (NHS KSF) and Development Review Process (October 2004).* DH, London.
Department of Health (2006) *Update our Health, Our care, Our Say.* MHSO, London.
Department of Health (2008a) *World Class Commissioning.* DH, London.
Department of Health (2008b) *Local Involvement Networks (LiNks).* http://www.dh.gov.uk/en/Managingyourorganisation/PatientAndPublicinvolvement/DH_076366. Accessed 2 June 2009.
Department of Health (2008c) PROMs questionnaires: terms and conditions. http://www.dh.gov.uk/en/Publicationsandstatistics/Publications/Publications PolicyAndGuidance/DH_091815. Accessed 6 May 2010.
Donaldson, L.J. (2000) Clinical governance; A mission to improve. *British Journal of Clinical Governance*, 5 (1) 6–7.
Donaldson, L.J. & Muir Gray, J.A. (1998) Clinical governance: a quality duty for health organizations. *Quality in Health Care*, 7 (Suppl) S37–S44.
Edwards, J. & Packham, R. (1999) A model for the practical implementation of clinical governance. *Journal of Clinical Excellence*, 1 (1) 13–18.
Garland, G. (1998) Governance. *Nursing Management*, 5 (6) 28–31.
Glacken, M (2004) perceived barriers and facilitators to implementing research findings in Irish practice setting. *Journal of Clinical Nursing* 136, 731–746.
Glover, D. (1999) Accountability. *Nursing Times Monograph.* Emap Healthcare, London.
Kitson, A. (1997) Using evidence to demonstrate the values of nursing. *Nursing Standard*, 11 (28) 34–39.

Long, A. & Harrison, S. (1996) Evidence based decision making. *Health Service Journal*, 106, 1–11.

Martin, V. (2000) How to manage, Part 6. Individual performance. *Appraisal Nursing Times*, 96 (21) 41.

May, A., Alexander, C. & Mulhall, A. (1998) Research utilization in nursing: barriers and opportunities. *Journal of Clinical Effectiveness*, 3 (2) 59–63.

Mayatt, V.L. (1995) *The CNST – How to Meet the Risk Management Standards and Reduce Financial Losses*. HRRI Conference, Paper Sedgwick UK Ltd., Edinburgh.

Mayatt V.L. (2004) (ed) *Tolley's Managing Risk in Healthcare: Law And Practice*, 2nd edition, LexisNexis, Croydon.

McCabe, C. & Timmins, F. (2006) *Communication Skills for Nursing Practice*. Palgrave McMillan, Basingstoke.

McCormack, B., Manley, K. & Garbett, R. (2004) (eds) *Practice Development in Nursing*. Blackwell Publishers, Oxford.

McSherry, R. (1997) What do registered nurses and midwives feel and know about research. *Journal of Advanced Nursing*, 25, 985–988.

McSherry, R. & Haddock, J. (1999) Evidence based health care: its place within clinical goverance. *British Journal of Nursing*, 8 (2) 113–117.

McSherry, R. & Warr, J. (2008) *An Introduction to Excellence in Practice in Health and Social*. Open University Press, Maidenhead.

McSherry, R., Artley, A. & Holloran, J. (2006) Research awareness: an important factor for evidence based nursing. *World Views on Evidence-Based Nursing 3*, 3, 103–115.

McSherry, R., Simmons, M. & Abbott, P. (2001) *Evidence-Informed Nursing: A Guide for Clinical Nurses*. Routlege, London.

National Health Service Institute for Innovation and Improvement (2009) Guest Editorial IN THE DRIVER'S SEAT: Using service improvement tools to drive up quality, drive out inefficiencies and drive down costs. http://www.institute.nhs.uk/nhs_alert/guest_editorials/July_2009_Guest_Editorial.html. Accessed 18 September 2009.

National Health Service Litigation Authority (2009) Risk Management. http://www.nhsla.com/RiskManagement/. Accessed 18 September 2009.

NHS Executive (1999b) *Health Services Circular 1999/154 Continuing Professional Development: Quality in the New NHS*. DH, London.

NHS Executive (1999c) *Health Service Circular 1999/053 For The Record: Managing Records in NHS Trusts and Health Authorities*. Department of Health, London.

NHS Executive (2000a) *Information for Health*. Department of Health, London.

NHS Executive (2000b) *Health Service Circular 2000/Caldicott Report*. Department of Health, London.

O'Neill, S. (2000) Clinical governance in action Part 4: communication. *Professional Nurse*, 16 (1) 816–817.

Pearce, P. & McSherry, R. (2000) Development: making it happen. *Health Care Risk Report*, 6 (10) 15–17.

Pennels, C. (1997) Nursing and the law: clinical responsibility. *Professional Nurse*, 13 (3) 162–164.

RCN (2000) *Clinical Governance: How Nurses Can Get Involved*. Royal College of Nursing, London.

Sackett, L.D., Rosenburg, W. & Haynes, B.R. (1997) *Evidence Based Medicine; How to Practise and Teach EBM*. Churchill Livingstone, London.

Scally, G. & Donaldson, L.J. (1998) Clinical governance and the drive for quality improvement in the new NHS in England. *BMJ*, 137, 61–65.

Swage, T. (1998) Clinical care takes center stage. *Nursing Times*, 94 (14) 40–41.

Oxford University (2009) Patient-Reported Outcome Measures (PROMs) http://phi.uhce.ox.ac.uk/home.php. Accessed 18 September 2009.

Walshe, K., Freeman, T., Latham, L., Wallace, P. & Spurgeon, P. (2000) *Clinical Governance: From Policy to Practice*. Health Services Management Centre, University of Birmingham, Birmingham.

Williams, C.A. & Heins, R.M. (1976) *Risk Management and Insurance*. McGraw-Hill, New York.

Wilson, J. & Tingle, J. (eds) (1999) *Clinical Risk Modification: A Route to Clinical Governance*. Butterworth Heinemann, Oxford.

Chapter 4

Applying Clinical Governance in Daily Practice

Rob McSherry and Paddy Pearce

Introduction

Chapter 3 explored in detail the key components of clinical governance and the systems and processes necessary for its success. This chapter builds on the previous chapters by offering practical examples on how to facilitate the application of the clinical governance framework at an organisational, team and individual level. To make the introduction of clinical governance easier it is important that any organisation, team or individual is clear about what clinical governance is and why it is important to the promotion of clinical quality and excellence in practice (Chapter 2).

Clinical governance is 'a framework through which NHS organisations [and the independent sector] are accountable for continuously improving the quality of their services and safeguarding high standards of care, by creating an environment in which clinical excellence in clinical care will flourish' (DH 1997). It emerges from this definition that the successful development, implementation and evaluation of clinical governance frameworks are associated with 'two distinct elements – the mechanistic element of ensuring systems are in place, and the more philosophical element of producing a culture in which clinical quality can flourish' (Haslock 1999, p. 744).

To advance clinical governance within the NHS and the Independent Sector, all healthcare organisations need to establish their level of quality as required by the Department of Health in the Health Service Circular HSC 1999/065 (NHS Executive 1999). To achieve these standards within any healthcare organisation a baseline assessment of their existing organisational systems and processes is required. The baseline assessment is necessary to reveal strengths and weaknesses of existing systems and

Clinical Governance, third edition. By Rob McSherry and Paddy Pearce.
Published 2011 by Blackwell Publishing Ltd.

processes so that a robust action plan can be developed to facilitate the development, implementation and evaluation of clinical governance. The baseline assessment should be linked to the Standards for Better Health (DH 2004) or other relevant agencies standards, i.e. Commission for Social Care Inspection (CSCI). As stated in previous chapters these standards for health and social care will be replaced by the Care Quality Commissions (CQC) requirements for registration in April 2010. The difficulty for many healthcare organisations, teams and individuals is, where does this process begin? A starting point would be to consider the CQC registration requirements as a guiding framework.

Introducing clinical governance into healthcare organisations

Given the importance that the government attaches to clinical governance, by making the healthcare organisations' chief executive accountable for the successful implementation of clinical governance structures in the pursuit of clinical excellence, it is easy to see why many of the leads for clinical governance are members of the executive board, i.e. Medical Directors or Directors of Nursing. The rationale for this is quite simple: clinical governance is about achieving high quality within clinical and non-clinical services. Therefore it is important that any strategy is led by a clinician who has the respect and confidence of his or her peers, along with an ability to influence, guide and lead fellow healthcare professionals through the change management process.

For all healthcare organisations the first step towards implementing clinical governance is the identification of individuals to be given the lead responsibility for taking forward the development, implementation and evaluation of a clinical governance strategy. Having identified the lead person responsible for the strategic development of the clinical governance framework, clinical governance committees (CGCs), healthcare governance committee (HCG) and or integrated governance committees (IGC) have been developed as subcommittees of healthcare organisations' executive boards. The CGC, HCG or IGC comprise senior members of staff representing various professional, human resources and managerial aspects of the organisation, with an overview of and responsibility for maintaining key components of the clinical governance framework, i.e. clinical risk, quality, performance management and professional development, as illustrated in Fig. 4.1.

Figure 4.1 describes the hierarchical relationships between the management levels, professional groups and the key components of clinical governance. Each tier of the triangle is responsible for their own practice and accountable to the next tier, for example the clinical governance

The dashed line illustrates how effective clinical governance is dependent on two-way channels of communication

Fig. 4.1 Management structure associated with clinical governance.

subcommittee is accountable and reports to the Trust board. Examples of how clinical governance has been introduced with various healthcare organisations are offered by Edwards and Packham (1999), Haslock (1999) and Starke and Boden (1999).

The CGC's initial task was to ensure that a baseline assessment of their organisation's capability and capacity to implement clinical governance was performed in accordance with the guidance issued with the HSC 1999/065. Today we would argue the CGC, HCG or IGC are responsible for undertaken the baseline and approving, implementing, and monitoring the effectiveness of healthcare governance subsequent developments plan resulting from the baseline. So what does a baseline assessment and development plan look like?

Clinical governance: What is a baseline assessment and development plan?

The original HSC 1999/065 guidance provides in annex 2 a matrix of the standards requiring action by NHS Trusts, Health Authorities, Primary Care Groups and Primary Care Trusts. These standards needed to be agreed with the NHS Executive regional offices indicating how the key

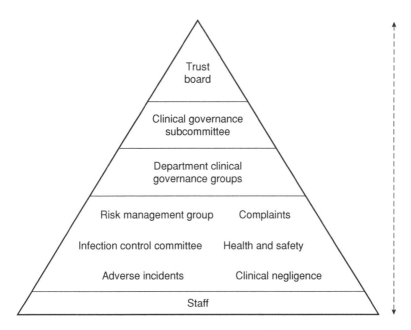

components of clinical governance were to be achieved for their respective organisations. A critical review of annex 2 reveals the main components of what a baseline assessment should consist of in demonstrating whether the organisation has the capability and capacity to deliver clinical governance. The annex can be summarised into four key areas as illustrated in Box 4.1.

The questions raised in Box 4.1 are synonymous with the information presented in Fig. 3.3 – the key components of clinical governance which describe in detail the systems and processes necessary for the successful development, implementation and evaluation of clinical governance. Figure 3.3 offers a framework that if used could provide organisations, teams and individuals with useful information regarding the initial clinical governance status and subsequent evaluations.

Furthermore the key components offered in box 4.1 could be used for the development of an integrated governance framework within any organisation.

Box 4.1 Components of clinical governance baseline assessments.

- Does your organisation have clear lines of accountability for the overall quality of clinical care and can this be demonstrated?
- Are there comprehensive systems for continuous quality improvement at all levels of the organisation?
- Is there a strategy for risk management and risk reductions?
- Does the organisation have an operational system for clinical performance management?
- Are there robust efficient and effective information systems for the collection and dissemination of information to influence practice?

Table 4.1 offers a checklist for undertaking a baseline assessment of clinical governance based on the information obtained from HSC 1999/065 (Lim *et al.* 2000).

From the information obtained from the baseline assessment as shown in Table 4.1, an in-depth action plan should be formulated building upon the strengths and weaknesses identified by the baseline assessment in measuring progress in advancing clinical governance in the areas of 'performance, developing infrastructures, staff and board development, planning and prioritisation' (NHS Executive 1999, p. 2). Essentially the action plan developed from the baseline assessment should have realistic expectations in relation to:

- Aims and objectives
- Goals
- Actions

Table 4.1 Baseline assessment checklist.

Standards	Full compliance	Partial compliance	Non-compliance	Additional comments
Risk management				
Risk management strategy and policies associated with clinical and non-clinical aspects of service		√		
Compliance with National Health Services Litigation Authority Risk Management Standards	√			Level 2 CNST
Systems for reporting and detecting: equipment failure		√		
Managing performance				
Systems for reporting and detecting:				
• Complaints	√			
• Clinical incidents	√			
• Untoward incidents	√			Consultant IPR
• Individual performance review	√			Introduced April 2001

Table 4.1 (*cont'd*)

Standards	Full compliance	Partial compliance	Non-compliance	Additional comments
Quality improvement				
Clinical audit	√			
Compliance with NICE and NSFs guidelines/recommendations		√		
Evidence-based practice		√		
Continuing professional development		√		
Quality information				
Clinical information systems		√		
Clinical outcomes data		√		
Comparative data		√		
Benchmarking			√	
Accountability				
Policies and procedures		√		All policies and procedures to be reviewed annually
Regular reporting to boards on efficiency and effectiveness of clinical governance	√			Monthly reports to boards

NB: Reference should be made to *Standards for Better Health* (DH 2004 or the CQC. 2009 registration requirements.) when completing this table.

- Time-scales
- Responsible individual(s)
- Monitoring and evaluation

These expectations should be shared with all levels of staff. Having shared this information with staff, directorates, wards or departments, they need to conduct their own local baseline assessment and formulate an action plan to achieve their specific and overall actions identified by the organisational baseline assessment (RCN 1998). This approach nurtures the philosophy embedded in the concept of clinical governance by involving all staff from the outset in creating an environment in which clinical excellence can flourish. The application of this approach reaffirms the notion that the outcome of the baseline assessment is a true reflection and representation of the organisational, team and individual levels, making future strategies for change easier to manage because clinical governance is everybody's business – a view echoed in the following statement:

> If clinical governance becomes some sort of parallel universe detached from day to day management and practice, it is likely to produce a resented bureaucracy that fails to deliver. It is only by embedding its principles and practice into everyday care delivery and organisation that it will succeed (Haslock 1999, p. 747).

To ensure that clinical governance does not become a bureaucratic 'nightmare' as alluded to by Haslock, staff must be fully informed of the managerial and strategic direction for the development, implementation and monitoring of clinical governance within the organisation, as outlined in Fig. 4.1. This could be done by having clinical governance briefing sessions, newsletters, governance seminars, learning and sharing from incidents which ideally involve staff in the early stages of the process. Activity 4.1 will assist you in ascertaining whether your organisation is successful.

Activity 4.1 is aimed at making you aware of how successfully your organisation's CGC, HCG or IGC communicated what and how clinical governance was to be implemented throughout your organisation. This stage in the process of developing clinical governance is essential in informing and involving staff before commencing the baseline assessment and subsequent development plan. Without staff's involvement in this process they are unlikely to understand and appreciate the importance of clinical governance at the clinical level; it will be seen to be owned purely by the senior management within the organisation. The clinical workforce may view this as yet another demand from government, construing it as not relevant to themselves or in the provision of services to patients. These misconceptions about clinical governance need to be tackled before

Activity 4.1 Clinical governance: baseline assessment questions.

During the early stages of a clinical governance baseline assessment it is essential that staff can correctly answer the following questions to act as a starting point for the development of clinical governance:

- Who leads clinical governance in your organisation?
- Is there a manager responsible for clinical governance?
- Who is the clinical governance lead for your directorate, team and department?
- Is there a clinical governance lead for your professional group within your organisation?
- Have you been involved with the baseline assessment at either organisational, team or individual level?
- Have you had any awareness training on clinical governance and how it may affect you and what you do?

Feedback is provided at the end of the chapter.

and during the baseline assessment. Failure to follow this approach could be the reasons why clinical governance in some healthcare organisations is not owned and viewed positively by the clinical and non-clinical staff in everyday practice – a perception confirmed by the following comment

> much of the machinery of clinical governance at an NHS Trust [and Primary Care Trust] level is now in place. However, it seems that clinical governance has yet to make a real difference at the clinical workface, and that changes in culture which it demands of healthcare organisations have not really begun to happen yet. (Walshe *et al.* 2000 p. 3)

Walshe *et al.* (2000) statement was correct at the time. Today the impact of clinical governance is emerging and is detailed in Chapter 7. Following the development of a managerial and strategic framework for the development, implementation and monitoring of clinical governance, as illustrated in Fig. 4.1, and the informing of staff about this framework and subsequent implementation of the clinical governance baseline assessment, the next step is the writing and developing of the clinical governance action plan. The aim of the action plan is eloquently articulated by the RCN in suggesting that the:

> Development plan shows how your organisation intends to build on what is working well, how it plans to improve, what it is doing less well and how it aims to fill any gaps. (RCN 2000, p. 7).

Furthermore, it is about sharing your successes and learning from when things don't work quite has well.

What does a clinical governance action plan look like and why are they necessary?

The clinical governance action plan should be developed in light of the findings of the baseline assessment undertaken by the CGC, HCG or IGC or nominated representatives. A format of how an action plan could be presented is offered by Garland (1998), RCN (1998) and Sealey (1999). The baseline assessment should highlight the strengths and weaknesses of the organisation in achieving the standards outlined in Table 4.1. The action plan should contain realistic targets directed towards improving infrastructures, performance and quality at organisational, team and individual levels. To some healthcare professions action plans are viewed negatively because they have predominantly been associated when things are not going so well. In this instance clinical governance action plans should be viewed positively and used as a guide for continuous quality improvements and in the sharing of good practices and performances.

Clinical governance action plan

Appendix 4.1 provides a detailed template of an example of a clinical governance development plan (for a local Primary Care Trust) broadly based on the key components associated with the clinical governance framework as highlighted in figure 3.3. The template provides a clinical governance assessment framework and development offering realistic aims and objectives, and identifies lead personnel to take responsibility within given time-scales for achieving each specific objective. The difficulty for some organisations, teams and individuals is relating the principles of clinical governance to their own specific daily practices (Malbon *et al.* 1998). Box 4.2 provides examples of case studies provided by other authors. The remainder of this chapter will use case studies taken from the authors' own experiences to demonstrate how clinical governance can be applied to our daily practices at an organisational, team and individual level.

Box 4.2 Examples of case studies relating to how clinical governance can be applied to clinical practice.

For examples of case studies relating to how clinical governance can be applied to clinical practice read:

Kausar, S.A., Rowe, M. & Carr, J. (2000) Avoiding medication errors and adverse incident: the way forward. *Clinical Governance Bulletin*, 1 (2) 4–5.

Northcott, N. (1999) Clinical governance No 1: organizational effectiveness–1. *Nursing Times Learning Curves*, 3 (2) 10.

Elcoat, C. (2000) Clinical governance in action: part 1 key issues in clinical effectiveness. *Professional Nurse*, 15 (10) 622–623.

Case study 1: Applying the principles of clinical governance to an organisation

A local hospital Trust has received a number of complaints from patients, and their carers, who have recently been admitted and discharged from the acute medical wards following a stroke (cerebral vascular accident). The complaints could be classified under the headings of poor quality care and poor communication.

Poor quality care

- Patients not having their privacy and hygiene needs attended to
- Development of hospital acquired pressure sores
- Failure to attend to nutritional needs
- Limited access to Allied Health Care services and rehabilitation programme
- Delay in home assessment and discharge

Poor communication

- Limited information about the patient's illness from medical staff
- Inconsistent information from the professional staff
- Inadequate capturing, monitoring and evaluation of patient safety incident data
- Failure to disclose information about patients' falls.

If each of these individual aspects of a complaint were reviewed in isolation it would be difficult to establish the severity of the problems associated with caring for stroke patients within this organisation. Having a clinical governance framework in operation within an organisation enables it to establish, understand and respond to clinical problems that are distressing to patients, carers and staff – a point echoed by Garside (1999):

> the big opportunity offered by clinical governance is the opportunity to change systems – to pull together different components and strands from the clinical and managerial worlds to improve things for patients.

In light of this statement let us explore in detail how the systems and processes associated with clinical governance apply to the case study as illustrated in Fig. 4.2.

Figure 4.2 illustrates how the key components of clinical governance can be applied and demonstrated in action at the organisation level.

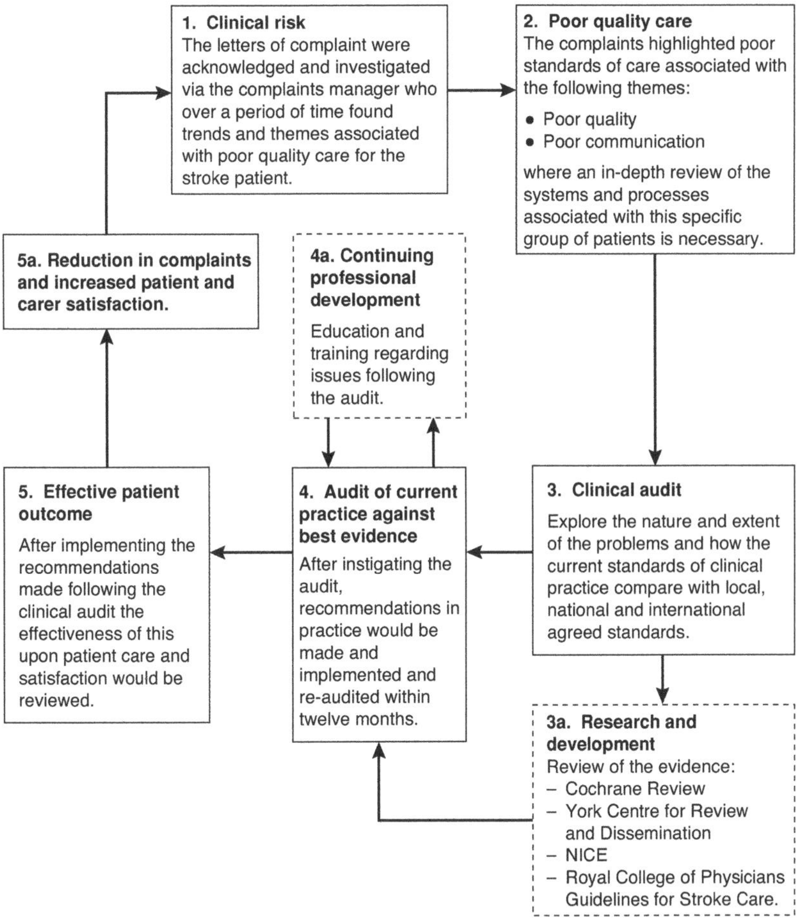

1. Clinical risk
The letters of complaint were acknowledged and investigated via the complaints manager who over a period of time found trends and themes associated with poor quality care for the stroke patient.
2. Poor quality care
The complaints highlighted poor standards of care associated with the following themes:
• Poor quality
• Poor communication
where an in-depth review of the systems and processes associated with this specific group of patients is necessary.
5a. Reduction in complaints and increased patient and carer satisfaction.
4a. Continuing professional development
Education and training regarding issues following the audit.
5. Effective patient outcome
After implementing the recommendations made following the clinical audit the effectiveness of this upon patient care and satisfaction would be reviewed.
4. Audit of current practice against best evidence
After instigating the audit, recommendations in practice would be made and implemented and re-audited within twelve months.
3. Clinical audit
Explore the nature and extent of the problems and how the current standards of clinical practice compare with local, national and international agreed standards.
3a. Research and development
Review of the evidence:
– Cochrane Review
– York Centre for Review and Dissemination
– NICE
– Royal College of Physicians Guidelines for Stroke Care.

Fig. 4.2 Applying the principles of clinical governance at organisational level.

The case study demonstrates how clinical governance offers continuous quality improvement by working in collaboration and partnership with the various departments and their associated systems and processes (Northcott 1999).

In this instance when the complaints had been investigated the main issues were about poor quality not related to individual clinicians but to the systems and processes that clinicians had to work in. An analysis of the complaints revealed two areas within the clinical governance framework that required urgent attention: poor quality and poor communication, particularly information gathering and disseminating. The application of the clinical governance framework to this situation enabled a full review of the current standards of practices and this was subsequently reviewed against the best available evidence, and recommendations made and implemented in light of the findings.

The overall outcome of this case study reinforces the need for reviewing untoward incidents [Serious Untoward Incidents and or Clinical Incidents] or failures that have a recurring theme or pattern at an organisational level based upon a systems and processes approach, rather than at an individual level. The outcome of the clinical audit based on the application of the best available evidence could make strong recommendations for the following:

- The need for a continuing professional development programme because the findings of the audit could have revealed a deficit in the clinical and management's knowledge with regard to best practices for stroke patients'/carers'/users care.
- The provision of a specialist stroke unit or designated rehabilitation area where patients receive high quality multidisciplinary care from specialist healthcare professions.

These points are more likely to be addressed as the recommendations are based on a thorough review of the current service provision using the clinical governance framework. A framework applied in this instance highlighted clinical risks, poor quality, and ineffective communications and information-giving and patient safety information data which, if not attended to, could lead to increased levels of complaints and loss of local public confidence in this healthcare organisation. The long-term impact of this poor quality service could culminate in low staff morale and subsequent high levels of sickness and absence, thus exacerbating this clinical situation. As this statement describes: a poor lead organisation with a closed culture equals a clinical disaster waiting to happen. In this instance the notion of accountability becomes everyone's business.

The principles behind this case study could equally be applied to evaluating the existing practices for teams and departments within Acute Trusts, Primary Care Trusts, Mental Health Trust, Ambulance Trust and in the Independent Healthcare Sector. The emphasis is on disseminating good or not so good practice – a point reinforced by Smith (1998) when describing the effects of the Bristol case (see Chapter 1) where poor practices, performances and a closed culture culminated in higher than expected mortality rates for children undergoing cardiac surgery. Similarly to the findings of the Rowan Ward (a mental health unit located in the North West of England, United Kingdom) enquiry by the Commission for Health Improvement (2003). In the later case the Healthcare Commission noted that the local PCT had failed to assure themselves of the quality of a commissioned service. Similarly, the Healthcare Commission (2009) Report of the Mid Staffordshire NHS Foundation Trust found systematic failures which lead to inadequate care and services.

Case study 2: Applying the principles of clinical governance to a team

Case study 1 highlighted how the clinical governance framework can be applied to the organisation-wide situation in addressing weaknesses in practice and performance. Case study 2 explores how clinical governance can be used in a positive way to assist clinical teams to continuously improve and evaluate the services they provide.

An orthopaedic ward in a District General Hospital with a large elderly population had higher than expected incidence of fractured hips (fractured neck of femur). This demand on the emergency services led to increased waiting times for elective orthopaedic surgery such as total hip and knee replacements. The situation was further exacerbated by the shortage of qualified nursing staff within the orthopaedic specialty to care for this specific client group along with a shortage of physiotherapists and occupational therapists to provide rehabilitative support. In this instance no reported clinical complaints were recorded via the incident reporting systems or the complaints procedures. Clinical governance was used in a proactive way to support the healthcare professionals, managers and patients in developing new ways of improving the service and in responding to staff's concerns of not meeting government waiting list targets for elective surgery. Furthermore, the issues associated with low morale resulting from a perceived provision of suboptimal care. Figure 4.3 illustrates the systems and processes associated with the application of a clinical governance framework to support a service improvement at team level.

Figure 4.3 shows how the clinical governance framework can be used to enhance the quality of a service at team level by the harmonising of the various key components associated with clinical governance. We acknowledge that waiting times for elective surgery have improved significantly (Pearce & McSherry 2006) however this remains a issue in certain specialities where there is a shortage of healthcare specialists (Boseley 2002). In this instance a *performance management issue* was detected via the feedback from regional offices, stating that the Trust's targets for elective orthopaedic surgery were not being achieved. Yet, the principle behind the case study could be applied to resolve other performance management related issues. A *quality issue* was evident from several points of view:

- The quality of life of elderly patients and their families is deteriorating while the patients are on a long waiting list
- Patients are older and sicker when they are eventually admitted
- Hospital length of stay is increased
- Waiting list becomes longer

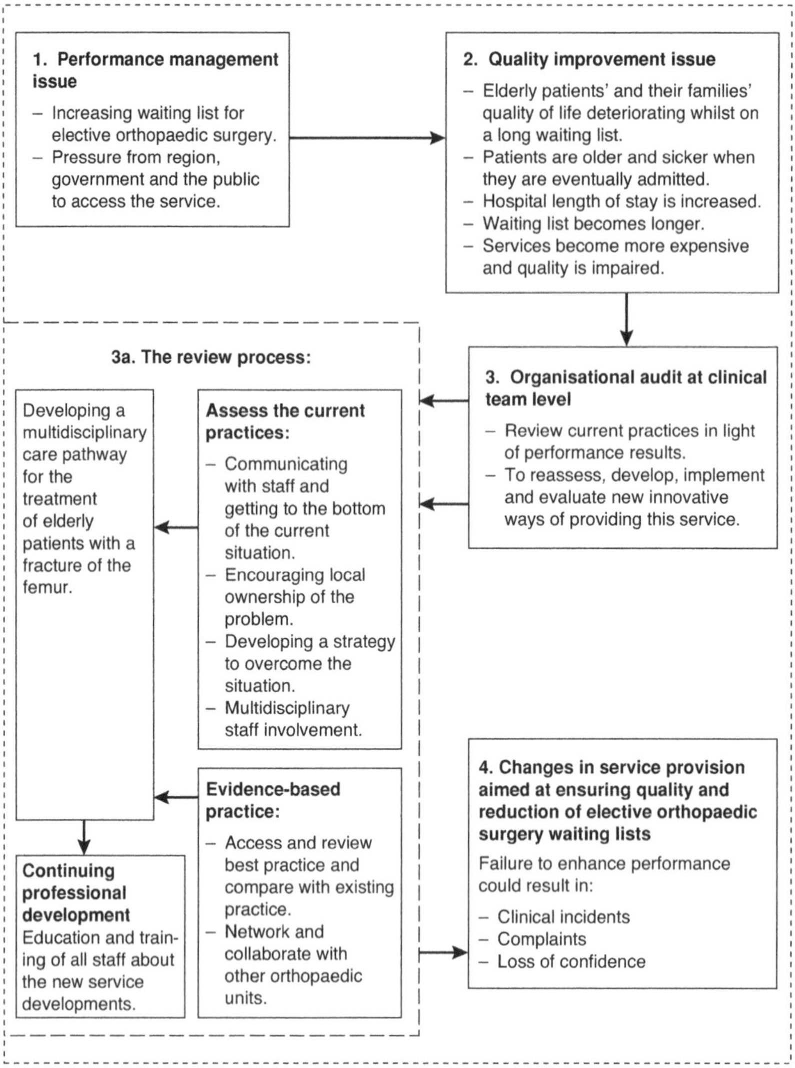

Fig. 4.3 Service improvements facilitated by the application of a clinical governance framework at team level.

- Services become more expensive and quality is impaired.
- Healthcare professionals become demoralised as a consequence of not providing the service to a level they would like to.

In light of the above performance and quality issues an *organisational audit* of the orthopaedics multidisciplinary teams was conducted to see where improvements in the current service provisions could be made. *The review process* required all staff to be involved so that local ownership and participation in the development of the new services were agreed by all members of the multidisciplinary teams. This proactive collaborative approach to continuous quality improvement is vital for the success or failure of any change – a challenge that is perhaps difficult and sometimes viewed as being unrealistic in today's NHS (Northcott 1999). The review process requires staff involvement in both accessing and reviewing best practices in the development and application of the new methods employed in resolving this clinical situation. To resolve the issues identified within this case study an integrated care pathway was developed and introduced after communication, collaboration and education of all the staff in ensuring the most efficient, effective and reallocation of resources.

In this case study, 48 hours after surgical intervention the patients are nursed on an elderly rehabilitation ward with the appropriate staffing levels to assist with the rehabilitation process. An integrated care pathway was instigated in this instance to 'ensure multidisciplinary processes of patient focused care which specify key events, tests and assessments occurring in timely fashion to produce the best prescribed outcomes, within the resources and activities, for an appropriate episode of care' (NHSLA Risk Management Website 2010). The integrated care pathway would ensure that an auditable trail of the patient's journey could be obtained and reviewed because 'the expected outcomes, frequently specified at different stages of the care pathway, are clearly described and any deviation or failure to achieve these outcomes or interim goals is quickly identified' (Benton 2000, p. 97). The drawback of this approach to providing care is that it can be viewed as cook-book health care.

The culmination of this approach ensures that the amount of orthopaedic elective surgery is increased because the beds are utilised more effectively. Failure by the clinical team to address this issue in a proactive way with the support of management and the clinical and non-clinical staff could eventually lead to increased patients' complaints or untoward incidents, making the need for change a reactive one not proactive – an approach that would certainly have an impact on the healthcare professionals working within this specialty area.

Essentially case study 2 demonstrates how using a proactive approach to implementing clinical governance can bring about improvements for patients, staff and management by the use of multidisciplinary collaboration partnerships in creating an environment and culture where all parties are involved from the outset.

As the saying goes, 'a problem shared is a problem halved'. How can we afford not to adopt this type of approach to promote continuous quality improvement?

The final case study in highlighting how clinical governance can be applied to the clinical situation focuses on its relevance to the individual healthcare professional.

Case study 3: Systems and processes associated with the application of a clinical governance framework at individual level

Case study 3 is adapted from the second case study in an article by McSherry (1999) in Health Care Risk Report that explored the value of practice and professional development in assisting an organisation and individual to use the principles of clinical governance in daily practice.

A 38-year-old woman complains to her local hospital on discharge. Following her admission on to the acute medical ward for treatment of painful joints, she says a senior healthcare professional (could be a nurse, doctor or any healthcare professional who undertakes adjustments to extend or expand their roles) was abrupt and insensitive when inserting a cannula into her right hand. This caused unnecessary bruising and discomfort because they tried several times to insert the cannula without success. The woman stated that it was not until a more experienced member of staff saw what was happening and took over this duty from the staff member that the cannula was inserted on the first attempt.

Let us explore in detail how clinical governance may assist in overcoming this clinical incident associated with an individual's practice. In recent years a nurse manager, on receiving this complaint, might have rushed into establishing how this had occurred and who was responsible for such an incident so that disciplinary procedures could be instigated. This reactionary approach to management does not bode well in the context of clinical governance that promotes a fair blame culture by the use of a proactive management style, as outlined in Chapter 3. Figure 4.4 illustrates how the key components of clinical governance can be applied to encourage the individual, team and organisation to learn and develop from this clinical incident.

In this case study the incident was reported via the clinical incident reporting system and was passed to the respective clinical manager for this directorate/ward to investigate and feedback the findings to the clinical risk management team for a response to be given to the client. To address and alleviate the situation the manager would discuss the incident with the individual and undertake a Strengths Weakness Opportunity Threats (SWOT) Analysis of the individual's strengths, weaknesses, opportunities and threats. This would pay particular attention to the incident and ensure that the healthcare professional had the necessary knowledge, skills and competence to perform the role of cannulation. If it was established that he/she lacked the competency or capability then a personal development plan (PDP) would be jointly agreed and written. This would incorporate regular monthly evaluations with the line manager. The plan could cover education and training in cannulation, shadowing staff and encouraging professional development in clinical information and skills.

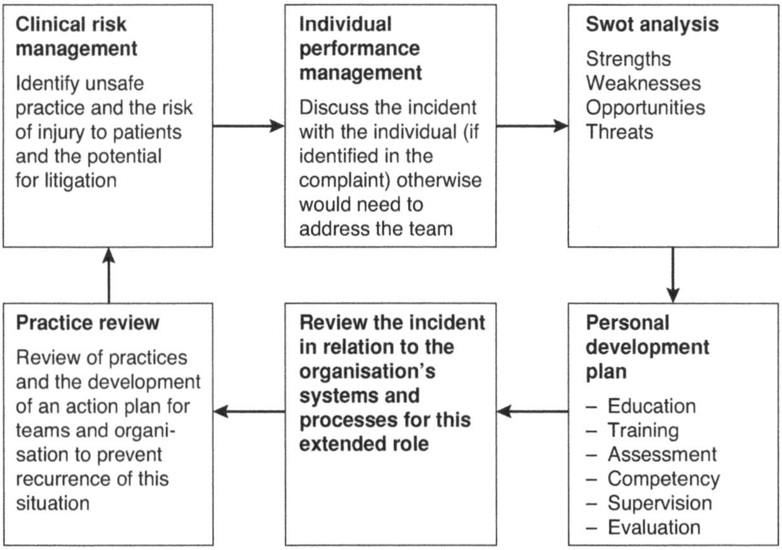

Fig. 4.4 How the key components of clinical governance can be applied to an individual.

The period for the PDP would vary according to the individual's needs. The professional may have been unaware of the discomfort caused to the patient for many reasons – pressure of work, not enough knowledge or training, incompetence, etc. The development and implementation of a PDP could be seen as an important tool to promote quality and standards of patient care and of effective clinical risk management for the following reasons:

- A clinical incident was reported (patient complaint) and investigated
- An assessment of the individual's performance was undertaken (knowledge, skills and competency) against established research evidence
- A personal development plan was written, implemented and evaluated under supervision
- The overall outcome for patient and staff should be improved standards and quality of care.
- Where possible the organisation should learn the lessons from this case to avoid recurrence.

An example of a personal development plan can be found in Appendix 4.2. In addition to supporting the individual to resolve the issues around weaknesses in practices and performance, a team or organisation could learn from this incident by reviewing their own practices and associated systems and processes aligned to the practising of intravenous cannulation. Case study 3 reinforces the concept of clinical governance at an individual level. It shows how practice and professional development can be enhanced under the key areas of clinical risk, performance management and quality improvement.

In summary, the case studies offer practical examples of how clinical governance can be applied to an organisation, team and individuals in the pursuit of clinical excellence. Case study 1 demonstrates how complaints about poor quality care can be a driver for continuous quality improvements at an organisational level. Complaints that are predominantly viewed negatively enabled a positive outcome to be achieved for the organisation by exploring and linking the key components of clinical governance. Case study 2 illustrates the determination of staff to improve their clinical services at a team level by collaborative working and partnerships, redesigning a new clinical service for the care of a specific group of patients and for healthcare professionals. This culminated in the development of an integrated care pathway for patients with a hip fracture, thus enabling more efficient and effective use of services and thereby improving the overall performance and management of the organisation. Case study 3 highlights how a proactive approach to the poor performance of an individual can be seen as learning experience to themselves, clinical teams and the organisation. In totality, the case studies demonstrate the clinical governance challenges in exploring how the principles can be applied across organisational boundaries (and sectoral frontiers) to ensure the overall management of the care pathway, as opposed to the organisational management of an episode of care.

Conclusion

In conclusion this chapter has outlined how healthcare organisations' capability and capacity to introduce clinical governance were initially assessed and developed by means of a baseline assessment and clinical governance development plans. The difficulties for some organisations, teams and individuals is in transporting the findings of either the organisational or local development plans into clinical practice. To assist healthcare professionals to overcome this concern, three practice-based case studies were presented and reviewed in relation to how clinical governance can be applied to these unique situations. The case studies systematically related how and where the key components of clinical governance could be linked to the various systems and processes of a healthcare organisation or Trust. Practical advice and guidance was offered throughout the case studies to enable the reader to apply the key components of clinical governance to the organisation, team and individual level.

Several themes emerge following the application of the clinical governance framework and the associated key components to case studies, which have the potential to inhibit or enhance the uptake of the goal of clinical governance – to promote continuous quality improvements and clinical excellence. Effective communication, collaboration and working in partnerships, and the development of a culture that values 'people' and their individual contribution to health care, are essential if clinical governance is to be realised in the reforming agenda of the NHS. We would argue that it is not the organisational structures alone that create a quality organisation, service or team; it is the aspirations, vision and values of the people who work within and for the origination. People not systems make things happen in practice.

Activity 4.1 Feedback – clinical governance: baseline assessment questions.

The initial stages of a baseline assessment should be concerned with ensuring that all staff can answer the questions in order to establish what is known and not known about the systems and processes associated with clinical governance within the organisation.

If you are unable to answer these questions we suggest that you require education and training on how clinical governance is being developed within your own organisation.

Key points

- Individual healthcare professionals should familiarise themselves with their local clinical governance arrangements and infrastructures for delivering the clinical governance agenda for their respective organisation.
- All healthcare organisations should have a baseline assessment and clinical governance development plan to develop, monitor and evaluate the impact of clinical governance to their own organisation.
- Clinical governance and its associated key components can be applied to three levels: the organisation, team and individuals.
- Clinical governance is everybody's business.
- A proactive management style and honest and open culture that values all staff, in seeking to learn from its mistakes in a fair blame culture is well on the road to successfully achieving the clinical governance agenda.
- It is not the organisational structures alone that create a quality organisation, service or team; it is the aspirations, vision and values of the people who work within and for the origination.

Suggested reading

Edwards, J. & Packham, R. (1999) A model for the practical implementation of clinical governance. *Journal of Clinical Excellence*, 1 (1) 13–18.

McSherry, R. & Pearce, P. (2004) Healthcare Standards: a critique of the Department of Health's National Standards for the NHS. *Health Care Risk Report* 10, 8 July/August.

RCN (2000) *Clinical Governance: How Nurses Can Get Involved*. Royal College of Nursing, London.

Sealey, C. (1999) Clinical governance: an information guide for occupational therapists. *British Journal of Occupational Therapy*, 62 (6) 263–268.

References

Benton, D.C. (2000) Clinical effectiveness. In: *Achieving Evidence-based Practice: A Handbook for Practitioners* (eds S. Hamer & G. Collinson). Bailliere Tindall, London.

Boseley, S. (2002) New Ideas hampered by shortage of specialist staff. *The Guardian*, 5 August.

Commission for Health Improvement (2003) *Investigation in Matters Arising from Care on Rowan Ward, Manchester Mental Health and Social Care Trust*. CHI, London.

DH (1997) *The New NHS Modern and Dependable*. Department of Health, London.

DH (2004) *Standards for Better Health*. Department of Health, London.

Edwards, J. & Packham, R. (1999) A model for the practical implementation of clinical governance. *Journal of Clinical Excellence*, 1 (1) 13–18.

Garland, G. (1998) Governance. *Nursing Management*, 5 (6) 28–31.

Garside, P. (1999) Book review. *Clinical Governance: Making it Happen* (eds M. Lugon & J. Secker-Walker) RSM Press, London. *BMJ*, 318, 881.

Haslock, I. (1999) Introducing clinical governance in an acute trust. *Hospital Medicine*, 60 (10) 744–747.

Healthcare Commission (2009) *Investigation into Mid Staffordshire NHS Foundation Trust*. Healthcare Commission, London.

Lim, J., Burton, T. & Bowens, A. (2000) *What Elements Should Be Covered In A Clinical Governance Development Plan?* Nuffield Institute for Health, University of Leeds & NHS Executive Northern & Yorkshire.

Malbon, G., Gillam, S. & Maysn, N. (1998 November) Onus points. *Health Services Journal*, 19, 28–29.

McSherry, R. (1999) Practice and professional development. *Health Care Risk Report*, 6 (1) 21–22.

McSherry, R. & Haddock J. (1999) Evidence based health care: its place within clinical governance. *British Journal of Nursing*, 8 (2) 113–117.

National Health Service Litigation Authority (2010) *Risk Management*. http://www.nhsla.com/RiskManagement/. Accessed 9 May 2010.

NHS Executive (1999) *Health Service Circular 1999/065 Clinical Governance: Quality in the New NHS.* DH, London.
Northcott, N. (1999) Clinical Governance. Effective staff – 2. *Nursing Times*, 3 (4) 10.
Pearce, P. & McSherry, R. (2006) From stars to health checks: looking towards the future. *Health Care Risk Report* 12 (3), 12–14.
RCN (1998) *Guidance For Nurses On Clinical Governance.* Royal College of Nursing, London.
RCN (2000) *Clinical Governance: How Nurse Can Get Involved.* Royal College of Nursing, London.
Sealey, C. (1999) Clinical governance: an information guide for occupational therapists. *British Journal of Occupational Therapy*, 62 (6) 263–268.
Smith, R. (1998) All changed, changed utterly; British medicine will be transformed by the Bristol Case. *BMJ*, 316, 1917–1918.
Starke, D. & Boden, L. (1999) Case Study – how to make it work. *Health Care Risk Report*, 6 (1) 18–20.
Walshe, K., Freeman, T., Latham, L., Wallace, L. & Spurgeon, P. (2000) *Clinical Governance: from policy to practice.* University of Birmingham.

Appendix 4.1
An example of a clinical governance action plan

As discussed earlier in this chapter, the clinical governance committee would establish the strategic direction for reviewing the status of the Trust's capability and capacity to achieve the standards outlined in annex 2 of the Health Service Circular 1999/065. Since the publication of the Health Service Circular 1999/065 many organisations have ongoing development plans to continuously improve the governance of the organisation. To comply with these standards a local baseline assessment were performed by nominated parties where a development plan was formulated outlining areas of good and not so good compliance. This process is ongoing. Following the formulation of the development plan the organisation should decide the best way to implement, monitor and evaluate the development plan. To do this successfully clinical directorates or departments need to develop clinical governance implementation groups or committees that are multidisciplinary, containing members from each of the main departments of the Trust, as well as key personnel such as clinical risk managers, goverence managers and other relevant parties. The clinical governance implementation group's responsibility is to oversee the development plan for their respective area by prioritising the work and producing a detailed project implementation plan for its completion. Below is an example of a written development plan that could support the organisation and directorate in achieving the standards outlined in HSC 1999/065.

To identify gaps in the present performance of the organisation and to bring these departments up to the desired standard the aims of the development plan could be as follows:

- To ensure all clinicians are involved in relevant evidence audit programmes.
- To ensure full participation in relevant national confidential inquiries, e.g. confidential enquiry into perioperative deaths (CEPOD).
- To ensure that the clinical standards of the national service frameworks (NSFs) and National Institute for Clinical Excellence Natural Institute for Clinical Excellence and Health (NICE) recommendations are implemented.
- To ensure that the clinical audit programme reflects the organisation's clinical governance agenda.
- To enhance risk management and performance systems and processes.
- To promote continued professional development of staff.

Clinical governance development plan year commencing April . . . to April . . .

Section 1: The patient as experience

STRENGTHS	WEAKNESSES
• Well developed systems of user involvement in Mental Health ○ Multidisciplinary service governance group ○ Regular patient satisfaction surveys • Patient involvement in CHD LIT group and Diabetes review group • PALS has been established • PCT Patient Forum has been established • Began the process of developing the Patient and Public Involvement (PPI) PCT policy and established a group to progress this agenda • Experienced and skilled staff • Regular patient satisfaction surveys carried out in Community Dental Services • Good results from CHI National Patient Survey • Few patient complaints • High levels of public interest • Lots of good practice inherited from predecessor organisations • Received focus award from DOH/BDA for second year running • *Nursing Times* Palliative Care Award	• The extent of other independent contractors' systems development is unknown • Less known – not systematically collated at a PCT level – between primary and secondary care

ACTION	GROUP/PERSON RESPONSIBLE	DATE
• To further develop PALS – regular audit to monitor the effectiveness of the service	Head of Corporate Affairs	Ongoing✓
• To Take part in the national patient surveys for PCTs and Mental Health	Head of Corporate Affairs	April/May✓
• To feed back results from the national surveys to staff and patients		
○ Presentation at staff briefing	Head of Corporate Affairs	June/July✓
○ Produce an article for *PCT World* (the PCT staff magazine, published on a monthly basis)	Head of Corporate Affairs	July✓
○ Place information on the PCT's shared folders (intranet)		
• To use the information gleaned from the national surveys to inform and influence how we deal with and involve patients and carers (action plan produced)	PPI Group	Dec✓
• To continue to use every opportunity to involve *patient and carers*	PPI	Ongoing✓
• To introduce a system to monitor pressure prevalence in the Community Hospitals	Head of Healthcare Governance	June✗
• To extend the regular patient satisfaction surveys in Primary Care and Community Hospitals	Head of Healthcare Governance	Sept✗
• Work to create positive relationship with Primary Care Forum	PPI Group	Ongoing✓
• To further develop a cohesive PPI strategy for the PCT	Head of Corporate Affairs	Sept✓✓
• To increase staff awareness of PPI including independent contractors by holding workshops and training sessions	Head of Corporate Affairs	Sept✓
• To implement the new Complaints Procedure for patients	Complaints Manager	June✓
• To provide information and training on the new complaints procedure to staff including independent contractors	Complaints Manager	June✓
• To further develop closer links with the Community and Voluntary sectors particularly with 'hard to reach' groups	Head of Corporate Affairs	March

ACTION	GROUP/PERSON RESPONSIBLE	DATE
• To consider PPI on all PCT committees and groups (Patient Forum members on RM & A & CG Sub-Committees)	Head of Corporate Affairs	June✓
• To actively seek patient involvement on each modernisation project	Head of Corporate Affairs	Ongoing✓
• To actively use information from complaints and PALS issues to learn as an organisation to improve the patient experience	Complaints Manager/Head of Corporate Affairs	Ongoing✓
• To engage with young people regarding their health issues (vulnerable (older and younger) people)	Public Health Manager	Dec
• To share information about Patient experience with local government organisations	Head of Corporate Affairs	Ongoing ✓(via
• To further develop the links between PALS and Patient Forum	Head of Corporate Affairs	Ongoing SPL)
• Patient experience of commissioned services		

Section 2: Use of information

STRENGTHS	WEAKNESSES
• Strong performance management culture – much information on services commissioned from acute providers and Ambulance Trust • Robust HR systems • Good access to IT and the internet at Headquarters • Robust IT infrastructure and rapidly developing data collection in Primary Care • Regular clinical auditing undertaken in Primary Care and shared with the PCT • Regular complaints information to the Board • Caldicott Guardian in post • New IM & T team appointed	• Limited access to IT and clinical information to community clinicians • Little information on patient outcomes • Weak systems and mechanisms to feedback information to staff • Information Governance limited knowledge

ACTION	GROUP/PERSON RESPONSIBLE	DATE
• Improve methods of making information more accessible to staff		
○ Use of Team Briefing	Communications Manager	Ongoing✓
○ Team Meetings	Communications Manager and Head of Healthcare Governance	(Meet monthly)
• Regular feature and articles in PCT World	Head of Healthcare Governance	Quarterly✓
• Carry out an assessment of current information available	Communications Manager, Public Health Information Officer and Head of Healthcare Governance	Sept✓
• Regular progress against implementation of the NHS IM & T Strategy	Head of IM & T	Quarterly✓
• Further refinement and development of a strategic approach to how we as a PCT use information	Communications Manager, Public Health Information Officer and Head of Healthcare Governance and IM & T	Sept✓
○ Establish a formal information group		Ongoing (group set up)✓
• Develop the concepts Knowledge Management Evidence Based Healthcare		
• Review IM & T development and strategy and disseminate widely	Head of IM & T	April✓
• Develop a Governance Section of the H & R PCT's website	Communications Manager and Head of Healthcare Governance	Sept✗
• Perform a baseline audit of Healthcare Records	Head of Healthcare Governance	March✓
• Provide training on Information Governance	Training & Education Manager	March

Section 3: Processes for quality improvement – risk management and incident reporting

STRENGTHS	WEAKNESSES
• Established Clinical Governance, Risk Management and Controls Assurance Sub-Committees • PCT has linked clinical and non-clinical governance via the concept of 'healthcare governance' • Small competent and skilled healthcare governance department established • Established 'Accident, Incident & Clinical Incident Reporting System', including near misses for all staff employed by the PCT • Community Pharmacy have piloted a drug error reporting system • Culture of significant incident reviewing developing in Primary Care	• Variable incident reporting in primary care • Newly established immature organisation • Only limited reporting from independent contractors

ACTION	GROUP/PERSON RESPONSIBLE	DATE
• To further develop and strengthen health and safety arrangements and policies (HSE Visit)	Head of Healthcare Governance	Sept✓
• To continually monitor and implement relevant Controls Assurance action plans	Head of Healthcare Governance	Ongoing✓
• To review Accident, Incident and Clinical Incident Reporting Policy and gain PCT Board Approval	Head of Healthcare Governance	March✓
• To ensure that PCT is able to report all clinical incidents to the NPSA via the National Reporting and Learning System (NRLS)	Head of Healthcare Governance	April✓

ACTION	GROUP/PERSON RESPONSIBLE	DATE
• To further develop the methods for feeding back summary information from the incident reporting system to managers & clinicians, including near misses	Head of Healthcare Governance	Ongoing✓
• To further develop risk management training programmes for all levels of staff within the organisation	Head of Healthcare Governance and Educ, Trg & Dev Manager	Ongoing✓ Jan✓
• To ensure 8 appropriate senior managers/clinicians undertake root cause analysis training provided by the NPSA	Head of Healthcare Governance	Mar✓
• To work with independent contractors to reduce clinical risks – offer/share PCT policies and procedures	Head of Healthcare Governance	
• Continue to work with community pharmacists to improve the drug prescribing and dispensing errors	Pharmaceutical Advisor	Ongoing✓
• To raise awareness of clinical risk management and incident reporting	RM & CA SC & Head of Healthcare Governance	Ongoing✓
• To hold a Governance Seminar focused on Risk Management and Learning the lessons from clinical incidents		Jan

Section 4: Processes for quality improvement – research and development

STRENGTHS	WEAKNESSES
• Have developed a Research Governance Implementation Plan • Several GPs with special interest in research • TARGET days encourage research based approach through the inclusion of targeted sessions • PCT is a member of a local Research Management • Head of Healthcare Governance is a member local Research Governance Scientific Committee	• Little experience of Primary Research

ACTION	GROUP/PERSON RESPONSIBLE	DATE
• To raise the awareness of R & D within the PCT – consider cost implications	CG SC	March✓
• Ensure good links to Acute Trust's R & D function	Head of Healthcare Governance	Oct✗
• To establish a PCT R & D Group	Head of Healthcare Governance	Sept✗
• To continually monitor and review the PCT's Research Governance Implementation Plan	Clinical Governance Sub Committee	Quarterly✓
• To establish a database of all research activity within the PCT	Clinical Audit & Effectiveness Facilitator	June✓
• To report regularly to the Clinical Governance Sub-Committee on research	Head of Healthcare Governance and R & D Group	Quarterly✓

Section 5: Clinical audit and clinical effectiveness

STRENGTHS	WEAKNESSES
• Well-established culture of clinical audit in Mental Health ○ Annual clinical audit programme ○ Regular meeting of most disciplines ○ Robust suicide audit • Good but limited history of countywide audit for GPs • Part of the countywide audit group developing NSF-based audits for CHD, diabetes and older people/stroke • Established collaborative CHD modernisation group, consisting of primary and secondary care staff focused on the CHD NSF • Employed a Clinical Audit & Effectiveness Facilitator responsible for progressing Clinical Audit & Effectiveness within the PCT	• Suboptimal development of activity/capacity • Protected time for development of audit programmes • Access to online resources in clinical setting • Limited capacity of clinical effectiveness and audit skills

ACTION	GROUP/PERSON RESPONSIBLE	DATE
• To develop a clinical audit programme based on the national imperatives i.e. NICE guidelines, the NSF and the LDP	Commissioning Team, Mental Health, CHD Modernisation Group, Prescribing Team Community Directorate	Ongoing✓
• Increase awareness and understanding of clinical audit by training & education	Head of Healthcare Governance, CGSC & ED & T Group	March✓
○ Provide training to departments and directorates		Ongoing✓
○ Develop training strategy with EDT group and Library service	Clinical Audit & Effectiveness Facilitator (CA & CE) ED & T Group & Library Service	Ongoing✓
• Aim to get 2 clinical audit projects from each clinical area per year	CA and EF	Ongoing✓
• Include input from Expert Patient Programme	CA and EF/PPI Group	Oct✗
• Establishment of Clinical Audit database	CA and EF	March✓
• To ensure the involvement of patients and patient groups in establishing priorities for audit work at all levels and all parts of the process	CA and EF	Ongoing✓
• To produce a clinical audit and clinical effectiveness strategy for the PCT to be approved by the Clinical Governance Committee	CA and EF	April✓
• To produce an annual audit plan for the PCT	CA and EF	June✓
• To provide the clinical governance sub committee with regular updates of progress with clinical audit	CA and EF	Ongoing✓
• To further encourage and facilitate clinical audit amongst independent contractors	CA and EF and ED & T Manager	Ongoing✓

ACTION	GROUP/PERSON RESPONSIBLE	DATE
• To link clinical audit in primary care with quality outcomes framework of the nGMS contract	CA and EF	Ongoing✓
• Establish a systematic approach to receiving, implementing and auditing NICE Guidelines	Head of Healthcare Governance, CA and EF Director of Public Health	Ongoing✓
• Continue to further develop an evidence-based culture	CA and EF	Ongoing✓
○ Clinical Effectiveness training day	CA and EF	Oct✓
• Baseline assessment of all primary care clinical areas, e.g. dentistry, physiotherapy, occupational therapy	Clinical Audit and Effectiveness Facilitator	Ongoing✓

Section 6: Complaints

STRENGTHS	WEAKNESSES
• Robust complaints system established with regular reports to the Board • Complaints manager in post • Robust policy • Meeting the NHS performance targets	• Not easy to link clinical incidents and other issues to complaints at present • Relationship – control of independent providers services e.g. NYED • No links to National Clinical Assessment Authority • Control of non PCT staff – Out of Hours Service post 1 April 2004

ACTION	GROUP/PERSON RESPONSIBLE	DATE
• To fully implement the new NHS Complaints Procedure	Complaints Manager	June✓
• To work in collaboration with other organisations to establish an integrated reporting and monitoring system	Incident reporting group & Head of Healthcare Governance	Ongoing✓
• To disseminate and share lessons leant from patient complaints throughout the PCT	Incident reporting group, Communications Manager	Ongoing✓
• To encourage and support primary care practitioners in the development of systems to manage complaints	Complaints Manager, Head of Primary Care, Head of Healthcare Governance	Ongoing✓
• To gather information regarding patient's experience of the complaints process in order to improve the system	Head of Corporate Affairs/ Complaints Manager	March
• To use the PCT prospectus to inform patients of system changes linked to complaints and the PCT's aim of local resolution nearest to the origin of the complaint	Head of Corporate Affairs/ Communications Manager	Dec✓
• To provide training on the new complaints procedure to a wide range of staff with emphasis on independent contractors	Complaints Manager	March
• To further develop links with partner organisations to aid the resolution of complex complaints	Complaints Manager	Ongoing✓

Section 7: Leadership, strategy and planning

STRENGTHS	WEAKNESSES
• Strong leadership from committed Board and managers • Introduced the concept of healthcare governance to converge clinical and non-clinical governance • Robust governance structure with clear lines of accountability • Non executive directors chair the Clinical Governance and the Risk Management and Controls Assurance Sub Committees • Director of Public Health and Head of Healthcare Governance are members of the local SHA clinical governance network • Strong communications policy • Communication manager in post	• The clinical governance structures and frameworks are still emerging

ACTION	GROUP/PERSON RESPONSIBLE	DATE
• Improved ownership from PEC and Board by participation in the NCGST Development Programme		
• To build upon the learning from the National Clinical Governance Support Team (NCGST) and National Primary Care Trust Development Programme (Nat PACT) development programme	PCT Board & Head of Healthcare Governance	Ongoing✓
• Continue to reinforce the visions and values of the PCT	Communications Manager	Ongoing✓
• To further develop links with PCTs in region	Head of Healthcare Governance	Aug✓

ACTION	GROUP/PERSON RESPONSIBLE	DATE
• To develop a clinical governance reporting template for clinical areas	Head of Healthcare Governance	Sept✗
• To raise awareness amongst the PCT staff and independent contractors by		
○ Holding clinical governance seminars	Head of Healthcare Governance	Jan✓
○ Training and education to clinical areas	Education & Training Group	Ongoing✓
• Disseminate good practice – via publication and conferences	PPI group	Ongoing✓
• Further development of PALS	Head of Corporate Affairs	Ongoing✓
• To conduct annual clinical governance visits to all GP practices – under the nGMS	Head of Healthcare Governance & Head of Primary Care	March
• To fully implement the recommendation of 'Assurance to the Board' and establish an integrated assurance framework	Director of Public Health, Director of Finance & Head of Healthcare Governance	March
• To ensure the PCT establishes a systematic approach to addressing the recommendations of the CHI & AC Review of the CHD NSF	Director of Public Health & Head of Healthcare Governance	May✓

Section 8: Staff focus

STRENGTHS	WEAKNESSES
• Open and honest culture • Robust and effective Joint Negotiating Committee (JNC) • JNC member on Trust Board • Staff appraisal scheme	• Communication remains challenging due to geographical spread of staff • Human resources training and development and organisational development strategies are being developed

STRENGTHS	WEAKNESSES
• Newly formed Education and Training committee • Regular staffing meeting • Team briefing • PCT World staff newsletter • High levels of staff involvement • IWL Pledge – Practice Award • Staff Handbook	• GP appraisal not fully bedded in – limited number of GP appraisers • New staff appraisal scheme not fully bedded in

ACTION	GROUP/PERSON RESPONSIBLE	DATE
• Review the results of annual staff survey – feed back to staff– ○ Team briefing ○ Clinical teams and localities	Head of Healthcare Governance & Head of HR	April–June✓
• Production of staff charter	Head of HR	June/July✗
• Establishment of a communication group to set, monitor and improve communication within and without the organisation	Communications Manager	June/July✓
• Establish a system to monitor CPD and link to PDP – linked to a corporate development strategy for CPD and PDP	Head of HR	March✓
• To develop/establish a development programme for middle managers	Head of HR & Educ, Trg & Dev Manager	March
• To further develop and expand HR services to address the needs of GP practices as/if required	Head of HR	June✓
• To further develop and refine the role of the Education, Training and Development Group	Educ, Trg & Dev Manager	July✓
• Perform a training needs analysis	Head of HR & Educ, Trg & Dev Manager	March

Section 9: Commissioning of patient/care/services

STRENGTHS	WEAKNESSES
• Robust performance management system for access to secondary/tertiary services • Developing good working relationships with local Hospital NHS Trust (main secondary care provider) • Good access data from primary care (GP) • Good access CMD • Head of Healthcare Governance member of Acute & Ambulance Trusts Clinical Governance Committees • Regular reports on Commissioning Services presented at Public Trust Board every 2 months by Director of Strategy and Commissioning	• Little information on the quality and outcome of care provided by service commissioned • Limited robust information of the quality and outcome of care provided in the community by GPs and GDPs

ACTIONS	GROUP/PERSON RESPONSIBLE	DATE
• To ascertain the clinical governance arrangements of secondary and tertiary care providers	Head of Healthcare Governance	June✓
• To continue to develop quality indicators/outcomes. Output measure for our main secondary care providers (linked to the LDP)	Head of Healthcare Governance and IM & T Manager	Ongoing✓
• Establish formal clinical governance/framework meeting/arrangement with main secondary care providers and relevant Acute Trusts	Director of Public Health & Head of Healthcare Governance	Ongoing✓

• In collaboration with other PCTs to agree a joint approach to understanding the clinical governance arrangements of major healthcare providers	Head of Healthcare Governance	Ongoing✓
• To agree a joint approach with other PCTs with regard to clinical governance performance of major healthcare providers	Head of Healthcare Governance	Ongoing✓
• To establish mechanisms to agree priority area of mutual benefit to the PCT and provider organisations	Head of Healthcare Governance	Ongoing✓

Staff designations

Clinical Audit and Effectiveness Facilitator–
Clinical Nurse Advisor, Mental Health Acute Services
Communications Manager
Complaints Manager
Director of Community Services
Education, Training and Development Manager
Head of Community Dental Services
Head of Corporate Affairs
Head of Healthcare Governance
Head of Human Resources
Head of Podiatry
Head of Primary Care
Information Management & Technology Manager
Mental Health General Manager
Pharmaceutical Advisor
PPI Group – Patient and Public Involvement Group
Professional Head of Clinical Psychology
Public Health Information Officer

Reference Dept of Health: *The New NHS Modern Dependable.*

Appendix 4.2
Example of a personal development plan

Note: This is a guide to how a clinical governance development plan may be presented and should be modified to suit your own individual, organisational or local requirements.

CONFIDENTIAL

HOSPITAL ....

DIRECTORATE ....

Name:

Position:

PERSONAL AND PROFESSIONAL DEVELOPMENT PLAN

Date: From .... To ....

Preceptor/supervisor ....

In order to achieve the compliance expected/required of a healthcare professional undertaking the role of venous cannulation within this organisation, the line manager (name) .... and staff member (name) .... performed a SWOT analysis of his current position on Date .... Time ....

Strengths	Weaknesses
• Confident • Competent • Time management • Enthusiastic • Committed • Adaptable to change • Relevant experience in taking charge of the ward	• Inexperience with cannulation • Had no formal education or training with regards to venous cannulation (see one do one)
Opportunity	**Threats**
• Access to personal development plan • Support and commitment to develop the role of venous cannulation • Support	• Clinical time versus personal time • Lack of time to attend courses on cannulation • Time on the ward • Perception of colleagues in light of the incident

Following the SWOT analysis, a personal and professional development programme was agreed. The agreement is as follows:

- to hold monthly reviews
- to document its progress after each session (see monthly review sheet)

- any new training/development requirements will be identified and added and dated as identified.

HOSPITAL . . . .

DIRECTORATE

WARD

Personal and professional development programme for

NAME . . . . **POSITION** . . . .

The following development plan has been discussed and agreed by

Name: . . . . **Date:** . . . . **Signature:** . . . . **Date:** . . . .
Preceptor

Name: . . . . **Date:** . . . . **Signature:** . . . . **Date:** . . . .
Preceptee

Identified training and development needs to be met by agreed competencies	Training and development method	Time-scale	Evaluation of training
To develop knowledge, understanding and skills associated with venous cannulation	To attend the in-house educating and training programme for venous cannulation To shadow a senior experienced clinician during cannulation To practise cannulation under the supervision of an accredited trainer To participate in cannulation audit within the clinical area		

Hospital . . . .

Directorate . . . .

Ward . . . .

Personal and professional development plan for NAME . . . .

Monthly review

Date	Progress	Signature

Chapter 5

Identifying and Exploring the Barriers to the Implementation of Clinical Governance

Rob McSherry and Paddy Pearce

Introduction

Chapter 4 offered practical examples on how the clinical governance framework can be applied to an organisation, team and individual in the pursuit of clinical excellence. For some healthcare organisations, teams and professionals the issues affecting the implementation of clinical governance are not associated with what it is and how the key components relate to practice, but in resolving barriers associated with the demands of a busy daily practice, the balance between improving quality and achieving increasingly difficult and forever changing targets, financial difficulties and a real and perceived lack of organisational support in developing staff. This chapter explores the potential barriers affecting the implementation of clinical governance and how they can be resolved by focusing on models of change, teamwork, collaboration, partnerships, leadership and cultural issues.

The potential barriers affecting the implementation of clinical governance

Barriers are defined as 'an obstruction, a fence or wall, anything that holds apart or separates' (Collins 1987, p. 67).

Clinical Governance, third edition. By Rob McSherry and Paddy Pearce.
Published 2011 by Blackwell Publishing Ltd.

Activity 5.1 Establishing the barriers to implementing clinical governance.

Reflect upon Collins' (1987) definition of barriers and make a few notes regarding what you think the potential barriers are to implementing clinical governance in your area of work.

Compare your notes to the themes in the Feedback box at the end of the chapter.

It would appear that Collins' (1987) definition of barriers is out of context when exploring the barriers to clinical governance within healthcare organisations. The definition appertains to the presence of physical presence which restrict movements. A critical review of this definition, however, shows quite the opposite.

Firstly, the word 'obstruction' refers to a blockage or anything that withholds or hinders the flow of something. If this term were linked to clinical governance, an obstruction would relate to anything that affects the quality of the vast array of systems and processes akin to its structures; for example, an obstruction in the channels of communication and information-giving between healthcare professionals and patients about preoperative risks and benefits associated with a certain procedure; or the failure to document an incident in the patient's healthcare records after a fall, where the patient/family complain about the incident asking for a full explanation several weeks after the event and no one can remember the event.

Secondly, a 'fence or wall' relates to boundaries, a term used frequently when exploring the relevance of clinical governance to healthcare organisations. Boundaries can be used as a means of protection or a barrier to be climbed. Within the context of clinical governance, boundaries should be used to safeguard the quality of the services.

Thirdly, 'holds apart or separates' suggests the need for dividing or keeping something apart for a specific purpose, whether this be for positive or negative reason. Similarities emerge when relating this to clinical governance and the associated key components that are separate by name but not in function; for example, the need for clinical risks to be detected so that clinical quality is improved or maintained.

It is evident from Collins' (1987) definition that barriers can be positive and negative in nature, which is of immense importance when exploring these issues within a healthcare organisation and the context of clinical governance. For example, the clinical governance framework could be viewed positively at organisational level because it provides a means to improve quality by developing its systems and processes, but for individuals in daily practice it may be viewed negatively because it is just another change without perceived relevance to their daily practices.

The barriers associated with clinical governance

> It is important in the implementation process within a Trust (or other related healthcare organisations) that the requirements for and the process of clinical governance be viewed with enthusiasm rather than scepticism. It can really only be satisfactorily implemented on the basis of a welcomed initiative with the potential for developing real improvements in quality of patient care rather than a political imposition. (Edwards & Packham 1999, p. 13)

For some healthcare organisations, teams and individuals this is not the perceived norm. Clinical governance is yet another 'thing' imposed by government in response to the poor media view of the NHS because of the high profile cases that have highlighted inadequate standards and practices – cases like those highlighted in Table 5.1.

Table 5.1 demonstrate high-profile cases that have undoubtedly negatively affected the public's confidence in the UK NHS, a confidence that requires rebuilding. Furthermore, Table 5.1 illustrates cross cutting and themes associated with the clinical governance components. To put bluntly, clinical governance 'is much more than a set of bureaucratic systems' (Harvey 1998, p. 8); it is a framework which is designed to help doctors, nurses, therapists and indeed all health and social care staff to improve organisational, team and individual standards and quality in pursuit of excellence in practice. To achieve the aims of clinical governance – reducing clinical risks, promoting continuous quality improvement and providing the best practices based on the best available evidence delivered by professionals who have the correct knowledge, skills and competence via a system of lifelong learning – a shift in attitudes and culture is needed to a positive view of clinical governance rather than a negative one. Cullen *et al.* (2000) states that we need to change the culture of healthcare organisation and to do this 'we need to unlearn some old habits and develop some new habits'. This view is supported by Davies *et al.* (2000) who states that we will need to 'change the way things are done around here' to unlock the true potential of clinical governance. The barriers affecting the implementing process of clinical governance are vast but not insurmountable, as outlined in Box 5.1.

Box 5.1 shows that the barriers to implementing clinical governance originate from internal and external sources which can affect the organisation, teams and individuals, as illustrated in Fig. 5.1.

The internal and external barriers affecting the implementation of clinical governance relating to the organisation or individual, as shown in Fig. 5.1, can be themed into several key areas as outlined in Fig. 5.2 and discussed here.

Table 5.1 High profile case demonstrating clinical governance issues.

NHS Sector	Case description	Issues linked to clinical governance components
Mid-Staffordshire Hospitals NHS Foundation Trust (2008)	Excess mortality rates and concerns raised over standards and quality of care with Accident and Emergency Department (HC 2009).	• Quality and standards • Communication and information • Clinical governance principles of transparency, openness and honesty • Accountability
The Neale Enquiry 2004	Related to a consultant gynaecologist who was found negligent for numerous surgical interventions resulting with unnecessary pain and suffering for his patients and their families (DH 2004a).	• Clinical governance principles of transparency, openness and honesty • Continued professional development and life long learning
The Bristol Case 1999	A consultant paediatric surgeon was found to have death rates for paediatric heart surgery significantly higher than the national average, and this only became known as a result of whistle-blowing (The Lancet 1998).	• Quality and standards • Communication and information • Clinical governance principles of transparency, openness and honesty • Accountability • Risk management and patient safety • Continued professional development and life long learning

Alderhay Childrens Hospital 2001	A consultant pathologist at the Royal Liverpool Children's Hospital, Alderhay, Liverpool, removed the organs of over 2000 children without the consent of their parents. As a result of an inquiry he was banned from practising in the UK, and all NHS Acute Trusts had to perform a census of their pathology department and list retained organs. The Chief Medical Officer issued guidance on post-mortem examination (DH 2001a).	• Communication and information • Research governance • Consent/confidentiality • Clinical governance principles of transparency, openness and honesty
Shipman Enquiry 2001	a general practitioner was convicted of the murder of 15 patients as a result of morphine poisoning (Ramsey 2001).	• Quality and standards • Communication and information • Clinical governance principles of transparency, openness and honesty • Accountability • Risk management and patient safety • Continued professional development and life long learning
Alitt Enquiry	a qualified enrolled nurse working in a paediatric unit was convicted of murdering four children and injuring nine others (MacDonald 1996).	• Quality and standards • Communication and information • Clinical governance principles of transparency, openness and honesty • Accountability • Risk management and patient safety • Continued professional development and life long learning

Box 5.1 The perceived barriers to implementing clinical governance.

- Lack of understanding
- Fear
- No clear vision
- It is nothing new
- It is a passing fad
- Lack of time
- Lack of resources
- Tool of the management
- Lack of support
- Poor information/no information
- Poor leadership
- Ineffective communication
- Lack of commitment
- No strategic approach to raising awareness, planning, monitoring and evaluation.

Note: This not an exhaustive list of the potential or perceived barriers to implementing clinical governance.

Internal	External
Individual • Lack of knowledge • Lack of understanding • Lack of confidence • Lack of ownership • Fear of what is about to be or is being left behind • Resistance to change • Ineffective communication • Information	**Individual** • Lack of support, i.e. peer, management or organisational • Lack of resources, i.e. personnel • Lack of time • Ineffective communication • Information
Organisation • Culture: openness, trust • Leadership styles • Lack of ownership • Management styles: – proactive/reactive – change management • Ineffective communication • Information	**Organisation** • Political pressure • Increased demand on already overstretched services • Increased performance targets • Public expectations • Increased litigation • Lack of resourcing, i.e. financial backing

Fig. 5.1 Internal and external factors influencing the implementation of clinical governance.

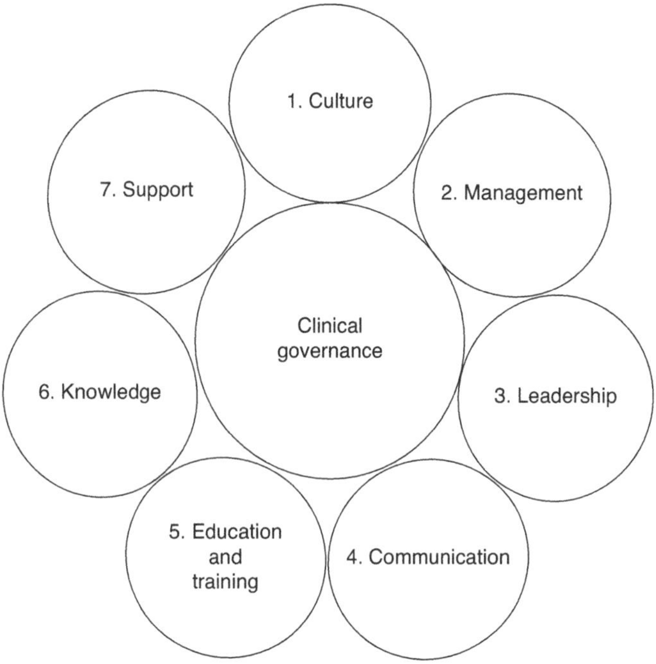

Fig. 5.2 Key themes linked to the barriers affecting the implementation of clinical governance.

Culture

What do we mean by culture? Culture is defined as 'the skills and arts, etc. of a given people in a given period; civilisation ... improvements of the mind, manners, etc. development by special training or care' (Collins 1987, p. 214).

During the late 1990s and early 2000s the word culture has become more prominent within the NHS, perhaps as a result of the many failures of healthcare systems, processes and the high profile professional misconduct cases, as previously mentioned in Table 5.1. A common theme that has emerged following the inquiries of past clinical disasters and investigations is the use of the word 'culture' or phrases like 'open or closed culture'. The questions posed by some healthcare professionals are:

- Why is creating the right culture important to the NHS?
- How do you go about creating the right culture for an organisation, team or individuals?

The Department of Trade and Industry (DTI 1997) suggest that an effective organisation recognises that shared culture, shared learning, shared

Table 5.2 Cultural barriers affecting the implementation of clinical governance.

Barriers	Rationale
• *Lack of openness*	• To encourage reporting of untoward incidents or practices. To state how you feel regarding a situation, whether it is good or not so good
• *Mistrust between employees and employers*	• To foster an environment where staff feel safe to whistle blow or voice concerns without retribution
• *Undervaluing staff*	• To create a feeling of confidence and pride in one's daily role and how that role relates to others, etc.
• *Not rewarding staff*	• Leads to low morale and inhibits the continuous quality improvements
• *Stifling innovation*	• Without nurturing continuous development the organisation and quality of care may not be developed and could deteriorate
• *Lack of transparency*	• Encouraging an openness where opinions within and external to the organisation are listened to

effort and shared information are the keys to high productivity and quality. For clinical governance to become a reality for any healthcare organisation, the cultural barriers outlined in Table 5.2 need addressing, as the rationale column suggests.

A healthcare organisation that is innovative, involving staff from all levels of the organisation and patients/carers, is an ideal foundation for the implementation of clinical governance an approach advocated by Haslock (1999):

> for clinical governance to raise standards in a genuine and lasting fashion it must be developed in a supportive, blame-minimising, educational atmosphere.

The challenge for some healthcare organisations, teams and individuals is how to develop this culture within their respective workplace. The starting point for addressing the questions associated with culture is to establish the type of culture within your present organisation or team. Hawkins and Shohet (1989) identify five types of culture, as outlined in Table 5.3.

Table 5.3 Types of culture (adapted from Hawkins and Shohet (1989) in Northcott (1999)).

Type	Key attribute	Preferred culture in achieving the modernisation of the NHS via clinical governance (the more asterisks the higher the preference)
Blame	A culture that seeks to address mistakes and apportions blame to individuals	*
Bureaucratic	An over-reliance on rules, regulations, procedures and policies at the jeopardy of individual personal judgement	**
Mistrust (watch your back)	An over-competitive environment that seeks to embarrass departments and individuals and stifles developments	*
Reactive (knee-jerk)	Short-term management plans and dealing with the immediate problem. No long-term vision	*
Proactive (learning)	Encouraging learning and development. Learning from mistakes.	*****

It is clear from Table 5.3 that a transformational culture is 'a construct that describes the nature of an effective culture' (Manley 2005 p. 62). In order for healthcare governance to occur a proactive transformational culture of learning is the most suitable for the implementation of a system of clinical governance. This is because an environment or culture that seeks to apportion blame only leads to secrecy, mistrust and a failure to report mistakes, with a knee-jerk reaction to resolving the incidents; for example, a healthcare professional administers the wrong medication to a patient, which results in no harm to the patient. The immediate response of management was to discipline the member of staff, who received a written warning on their personal file – a classic case of reactive knee-jerk culture that actively seeks to apportion blame because of failure to adhere rigidly to policy and procedure. This example

Table 5.4 The Manchester Patient Safety Framework (MaPSaF).

A	**Pathological:** organisation with a prevailing attitude of 'why waste our time on safety' and as such, there is little or no investment in improving safety
B	**Reactive:** organisations that about safety after an incident has occurred
C	**Bureaucratic:** Organisations that are very paper-based and safety involves ticking boxes to prove to auditors and assessors that they are forced on safety
D	**Practice:** organisations that place a high value on improving safety, actively invest in continuous safety improvements and reward staff who raise safety-related issues
G	**Generative:** the nirvana of all safety organisations in which safety is an integral part of everything that they do. In a generative organisation, safety is truly in the hearts and minds of everyone, from senior manages to front line staff.

Reprinted with kind permission from the University of Manchester (2006).

demonstrates the element of culture that is bureaucratic, reactionary and closed, by blaming individuals.

Alternatively, in an open learning or proactive culture the incident would have been dealt with by exploring and establishing the facts before apportioning blame, with the systems and processes reviewed before any action was taken against the individual. This approach treats the whole incident as a learning opportunity for the individual and the organisation and where possible offers support, if needed, to the individual and patient concerned. The lessons learned from the incident are disseminated throughout the organisation, in an anonymous way to avoid naming, blaming and shaming of individuals, to avoid recurrence of this type of event. The NPSA publication 'The Manchester Patient Safety Framework (MaPSaF) (2006) offers a typology of safety cultures Table 5.4 which complement the works Hawkins & Shohet (1989) outlined in Table 5.4. The framework by Parker and Hudson (2001), builds upon the work of Westrum (1992).

It is evident from Tables 5.1–5.3 that for healthcare governance to succeed, an environment is necessary that is open, honest, trusting and willing to learn from its mistakes and share good practices. The preferred culture to promote this type of environment is that of a 'transformation and constructive culture', a culture that:

- Promotes learning
- Learns from experiences and mistakes

- Communicates to all
- Collaborates between all levels of the organisation
- Rewards, values and develops staff at all levels
- Genuinely committed to the continuous improvement of patients safety and experiences of services
- Values diversity and treats all as equal partners
- Committed to Continued Professional Development and Life Long Learning of staff
- Listens and responds to feedback from services users and staff

This type of open or transparent culture takes 'time, and requires working for collaborative results rather than relying upon domination or compromise as a quick fix' (Northcott 1999, p. 10). Some organisations will require a cultural change to successfully implement clinical governance. This will not be easy and will require careful sustained management and effective leadership.

Management

The management style of a healthcare organisation will have a significant impact on how clinical governance is perceived and implemented. Management and leadership go hand in hand but there is a difference between the two. Marquis and Hutson (2000) suggest that management is about guiding and directing staff and resources and is concerned with having the power and legitimate authority for particular tasks and duties. Essentially management is primarily concerned with outcomes and the manipulation of resources to achieve the desired outcome(s). For example, in relation to clinical governance the chief executives of healthcare organisations are accountable to parliament for the implementation of the clinical governance framework, ensuring clinical quality along with meeting financial and performance targets – targets such as those outlined in the Care Quality Commission Regulatory Requirements and Care Quality Commission Periodic Review (CQC 2009) [which will supersede the Standards for Better Health (DH 2004b) and the Annual Health Check (HC 2005) from April 2010] and those existing targets such as patients been seen in the Accident and Emergency department within 4 hours of arrival; to be seen by a consultant within 13 weeks from the time of GP referral. These are all standards that require achievement through the process of delegation to other personnel within the organisation.

Management in this instance is about the transferring of roles and responsibilities to a specified team or individual for achieving the specific standards or desired aims and objectives. This collaborative and participative approach to management is the type that encourages a shared responsibility and ownership of what the organisation is trying to achieve. This is an essential attribute in the development, implementation, monitoring and evaluation of clinical governance, where the success of the systems and processes as outlined in Chapters 3 and 4 is strongly associated with the specific management style of the lead for that part of the service. For example, if the manager or lead clinician is autocratic and not prepared to listen to the opinions of others, this will have a detrimental effect on advancing the quality improvement programme.

Previously in the NHS, effective management was valued more than good leadership. 'In difficult times, people need leadership as well as management' (Stewart 1996, p. 3) – an approach advocated within the NHS of today in addressing the factors that have led to the introduction of clinical governance and in developing new and creative ways of implementing the key systems and processes akin to clinical governance. In this instance management is crucial in both highlighting key leaders to take on the roles and responsibilities for advancing clinical governance and in empowering them to do this effectively without managerial interference. The NHS Institute for Innovation and Improvement (2009) provide a variety of information and resources on effective management and leadership styles. So what is the preferred management style for achieving clinical governance?

Management styles and clinical governance

Several theories have influenced the management of the NHS (Marquis & Hutson 2000). These can be categorised into three broad headings that have some degree of applicability to the implementation of clinical governance because of the nature of the management style used (see Table 5.5).

It is evident from Table 5.5 that for clinical governance to be successfully implemented a combination of the three main management styles need to be applied at organisation and team levels. Each organisation or team should consider what their current management style is and what is the best way forward for them in managing clinical governance for the future.

The difficulty for some healthcare organisations and staff is not in eliciting what the preferred management style is or ought to be, but in overcoming the barriers associated with managing change effectively. For some healthcare professionals clinical governance is a challenging concept that is associated with the reviewing of existing and the development of new systems and processes requiring change at all levels of the organisation. To this end the success of clinical governance will depend on how this change is managed. The following sections on change management and reaction to change are based on McSherry and Simmons (2001), with

Table 5.5 Management styles and their applicability to clinical governance.

Theory	Description	Applicability to clinical governance
Scientific management	• Based on scientific principles • Efficient and effective use of resources • Having the appropriate staff and qualifications • Retaining and developing the staff • Valuing and rewarding staff • Cooperative relationships between managers and personnel	This management style is suited to the development of clinical governance because it links nicely to the notion of performance management. Performance management is associated with the continuous development and rewarding of staff.
Management functions	• Planning • Commanding • Controlling • Coordinating • Organising • Staffing • Directing • Reporting	This type of management style is essentially related to the core aspects of the clinical governance framework because it fits in with almost all of the key components. For example, command and control are associated with 'accountability'. Staffing and reporting are associated with performance management and clinical risk. The planning and coordinating are related to quality improvement.
Human relationships management	• Involving staff • Valuing staff • Staff participation • Involved and shared decision-making	This management style pertains to the humanistic element of clinical governance and the notion of working in teams, sharing and learning from each when things go well or not so well, along with the involvement of the patients who are viewed as an essential asset when developing clinical governance.

kind permission of Routledge, an imprint of Taylor & Francis Publishing Group.

Change management

Change is a complex process in which barriers are inherent, threatening the successful implementation of clinical governance. Utilising a change model can help guide the change process and help to reduce obstacles which may be encountered. Lewin (cited in Allen 1993) proposes a change model, the 'Force Field Theory', that has three fundamental stages – unfreezing, moving, refreezing – that could be useful when exploring the potential effects of introducing clinical governance within an organisation or team or for an individual.

Unfreezing

For change to occur, individuals need to recognise that there is a need for change. Lewin suggests that for unfreezing to occur there is a need to understand the driving and restraining forces that exist. For example, a driving force may be the limited availability of information to support a change in practice and the restraining forces could be negative attitudes from the staff about this aspect of not informing them what is going on. This is a potentially huge barrier to clinical governance, where staff are expected to operate within the systems and processes but have not been informed about them or what their roles and responsibilities are within them. Whilst these forces remain in balance the situation will remain in the status quo. Unfreezing of a situation can occur when driving forces are increased and restraining forces decreased.

Moving

This is where the organisation, team or individual begins to explore and examine the change or begins to accept or adjust to the changes being implemented. Teamwork needs to be nurtured and the emergence of key roles and responsibilities within the team highlighted. For clinical governance to work effectively staff need to be informed and involved with the change processes. Management therefore has a duty and responsibility in ensuring these actions occur.

Refreezing

Refreezing often occurs after a time, when the change has been accepted within the organisation or team and the individual staff settle back into

Table 5.6 Four main reasons for resisting change (adapted from Kotter and Schlesinger (1979) in McSherry *et al.* (2001)).

Type	Description
Parochial self interest	Where individuals may resist because they fear they may lose something they value as a result of the change.
Misunderstanding and lack of trust	Individuals often resist change because they do not understand its implications and perceive it might cost them more than they have to gain. This may occur where there is trust lacking between the person initiating the change and the workforce.
Different assessments	Individuals may assess the situation differently from those initiating the change and see more costs than benefits as a result, not only for themselves but for the organisation as a whole.
Low tolerance for change	Individuals may fear they will not be able to develop the new skills or behaviour needed after the change.

a functional unit, where key roles and responsibilities are adopted, supported and communicated to and from each other.

Having decided upon the model of change to be used, it is essential to be aware of how individuals may react or respond to the plans to implement the clinical governance frameworks.

Reaction to change

Most healthcare professionals find change disruptive and by merely exposing the flaws of a particular practice or presenting research findings to support the rationale for change, you will still most likely face resistance. While individuals may resist, different people will respond differently. There are four main reasons why people resist change, as shown in Table 5.6.

The potential varied responses by individuals to a change are vast but should not be overlooked when implementing change on a scale as large as that required for the successful implementation of clinical governance. Managers should try and establish the views and opinions of the organisation, team and individuals about the levels of tolerance, misunderstanding and interest in clinical governance so that the barriers to change can be avoided. The combination of effective management with leadership may help this process, as will be explored in the next section.

Leadership

Many people confuse management and leadership. Before we can proceed we need to understand the differences and relationships between leadership and management. This was eloquently described by Field Marshall Slim:

> There is a difference between leadership and management. Leadership is of the spirit, compounded of personality and vision; its practice is an art. Management is of the mind, a matter of accurate calculation. . .its practice is a science. Managers are necessary; leaders are essential. (Slim 1996 in Stewart 1996)

As mentioned in the previous section, managers are essential for the efficiency and effectiveness of an organisation and team. However, this is not to say that all good managers show the attributes that make successful leaders. For clinical governance to work we need leaders who can 'make others feel that what they are doing matters and hence make them feel good about their work' (Stewart 1996, p. 4). Mullally (2001) advances Stewart's (1996) works about leaders by incorporating the need for a moral and ethical dimension to leadership. This notion of empowering, involving and valuing staff is fundamental in developing the culture in which clinical governance will operate effectively.

The essential attributes of an effective clinical leader are that he or she is:

- a visionary
- a communicator
- a facilitator
- an advocator
- a critical thinker
- a doer
- an evaluator
- respectable
- knowledgeable
- tactful
- a motivator
- considerate
- ethical
- trustworthy
- credible

A clinical leader will utilise these essential attributes to influence and develop the organisation, team and individuals by the execution of a specific leadership style, which can be summarised into four main types, as illustrated in Table 5.7.

Table 5.7 describes how a transformational and democratic leadership style is potentially the most suited to implementing and evaluating a clinical governance framework. The issue for some organisations, teams and individuals is in establishing their leadership traits and how to address them. Table 5.8 offers examples of personality types (based on Allen (1993) and Lancaster and Lancaster's (1982) adaptation of Rogers and Shoemaker's example of personality types, used in McSherry and Simmons (2001)), with their traits and applicability to clinical governance.

Table 5.7 shows that the innovators would come out top for supporting the implementation of clinical governance. However it is important to mention here that an organisation or team requires a combination and harmonisation of all of these personality types to achieve success. It would be impossible to develop a service if all involved were laggards or rejecters; likewise, if everyone were innovators who were never really challenged about their ideas or introductions of new systems and processes, this could result in advancing practices based on a minority opinion. To advance this work the NHS Leadership Qualities Framework (NHS Leadership Centre 2002) offers five personal qualities of leaders that are useful when introducing clinical governance. These are as follows:

1. Self-belief
2. Self-awareness
3. Self-management
4. Drive for improvement
5. Personal integrity

When considering introducing or changing systems, processes associated with healthcare governance it is important to consider personality traits and qualities. The methods or changes advocated may or may not be the best way on this occasion. It is about finding what is best for the team or individuals. The way forward in exploring the issues associated with implementing clinical governance is about seeking the views and opinions of the staff. To ensure this occurs effectively, efficient channels of communication need to be effectively operated.

Communication

As previously mentioned in Chapter 3, 'communication seems to be about an interaction where two or more people send and receive messages, and in the process both present themselves and interpret the other' (McSherry 1999, p. 198). McSherry's quotation about communication relates to the

Table 5.7 Leadership style and applicability to clinical governance. (Adapted from Marquis and Hutson (2000).)

Theory	Description	Applicability to clinical governance
Authoritarian	Strong control • Gives commands • Communicates downwards only • Does not involve others in decision-making • Apportions blame	This type of leadership is destructive and inappropriate for the implementation of clinical governance. The whole style is at variance with the openness and sharing of clinical governance philosophy.
Democratic	• Less control • Directs by guidance • Two way process of communication up and down • Shared decision-making • Uses constructive criticism	This is the preferred leadership style for implementing clinical governance. It offers a strong vehicle for breaking down the barriers by the development of a collaborative, empowering and trusting culture based on a bedrock of communication and partnership.
Laissez-faire	• Little control • Limited direction • Communicates well • Devolves decision-making • Group orientated • Does not criticise	This style, whilst containing some elements central to the development of a clinical governance culture, is not without its limitations. Constructive criticism is necessary with the clinical governance framework.
Transformational	Interactive collaborative relationship associated with having the synergy to share the vision, lead the team and engaging the various team members.	Clinical governance is dependent on integration, collaboration and interdependent on the various systems and processes including people.

Table 5.8 Personality type traits. (Adapted from McSherry and Simmons (2001).)

Personality type	Personality traits	Applicability to clinical governance (the more asterisks, the more applicable)
Innovators	Curious, enthusiastic and eager	*****
Early adopters	Moderately enthusiastic, well-established group members, with high self-esteem. (Do not usually introduce radical/controversial ideas.)	****
Early majority	Accept the innovation just before the majorities do	***
Late majority	View the innovation with scepticism, do not actively resist	**
Laggards	Suspicious of change, discourage others by their negative attitude	*
Rejecters	Openly reject changes and encourage others to do so	*

need for a system of clinical governance because, 'without clear communication, it is impossible to give care effectively, make decisions with clients and families, protect clients from threats to well-being, coordinate and manage client care, assist the client in rehabilitation, offer comfort, or teach' (Potter & Perry 1993, p. 24). Effective communication is an integral ingredient for the success or failure of clinical governance. It is of paramount importance in ensuring effective communications between and within:

- The various systems and processes associated with the key components akin to clinical governance
- Individual healthcare professionals both clinical and non-clinical
- Organisations such as Primary Care Trusts, Strategic Health Authorities, Acute Trusts, Foundation Trust, Commissioning PCTs
- National Institute of Clinical Excellence, Care Quality Commission
- Department of Health
- Professional regulating bodies
- Non-statutory organisations
- Voluntary organisations.

A failure in communication between or within these organisations, teams or individuals could result in complaints about health care which are in the main linked to a failure in communications associated with 'staff attitudes, poor inter-team communication or lack of information for patients' (O'Neill 2000, p. 817). For the systems and processes associated with clinical governance to work in harmony, it is vital to have a culture that encourages open channels of communication between and within all levels of the organisation, teams and individuals. Failures to actively encourage honesty, openness and 'freedom of speech' contradict the philosophy behind clinical governance of promoting an environment where clinical excellence in practice will flourish. 'Whistle blowing' and the reporting of poor practices, performance or competencies associated with the systems, processes or individuals should be encouraged via open two-way channels of communication between all levels of the organisation.

Communication can be enhanced and improved in the clinical environment by:

- Sharing of goals
- Information
- Learning
- Roles and responsibilities.

In this way a culture based on integrated teamworking, partnerships and mutual collaboration becomes the norm. Clinical governance is not designed to work in a unidisciplinary manner; it needs teams and the individuals within the teams to collaborate, reliant on the efficiency and effectiveness of the communications processes.

Health care, and indeed clinical governance, is team-based, relying on the 'direct or indirect support and influences of others, either from their own or other professions or work groups' (Northcott 1999).

This point is highlighted by the NHS Circular 1999/065 where multidisciplinary and multiagency collaboration is viewed as an essential component for improving the efficiency and effectiveness of the health service. Effective team working and multidisciplinary or multiagency approaches to care delivery are only truly effective where communication is continuous and seamless. For example, it would be fair to state that a patient's recovery from stroke is interdependent on multidisciplinary collaboration and effective communications, not individual practices. For clinical governance to function efficiently and effectively healthcare professions need to have the ability to coordinate patient/carers' care by passing information to and fro within the multidisciplinary team, a skill which requires effective management and leadership qualities.

If we find it difficult to communicate effectively with each other and with patients, what can one expect to find when it comes to reviewing standards and when faced with the challenge of implementing clinical governance into organisation, team or individual practices? For clinical governance to succeed it becomes evident that communication is of paramount importance as it is the unifying factor that crosses through all the key components. Communications should be based on the following principles:

- Appreciation and understanding of individual roles and responsibilities
- Open channels of communication between and within the organisation, teams and individuals
- An ability to:
  - actively listen
  - express concerns
  - trust
  - work in teams
  - develop partnerships
  - collaborate
  - respond and act.

To achieve effective communications in supporting the implementation and evaluation of the clinical governance framework the organisation, teams and individuals need to be adequately informed. The latter can only be achieved by offering the appropriate education and training.

Education and training

The education and training needs of healthcare professionals should be considered on a NHS-wide basis to inform and educate staff within all levels of the organisation about clinical governance. The education and training of all NHS personnel should be based on a 'need to know basis' where the appropriate information is provided about how clinical governance affects them and their role. To ensure that this happens, the employee and employer have a mutual responsibility to ensure that education and training are provided at a local level. Further information on education and training is detailed in Chapter 8.

Knowledge

To ensure that all healthcare staff have sufficient knowledge and understanding of clinical governance, the education and training should be targeted to specific audiences with relevant aims and objectives that relate to and reflect the realities of their clinical or non-clinical practice. Further information is provided in Chapter 8.

To foster this approach to shared learning and problem solving relating to the development, implementation and monitoring and evaluation of clinical governance, healthcare organisations, teams and individuals need to be supported.

Support

The success of clinical governance will depend on the support and resources given within the various levels of the NHS to implement such a wide-ranging system. We believe that the support falls into two categories, internal and external, as highlighted in Fig. 5.3.

Figure 5.3 shows how the supporting infrastructures for the successful implementation of clinical governance depend on collaboration, partnerships and adequate levels of resourcing at organisational, team and individual level and effective communication. The support is not just about financial backing but the physical releasing of staff to develop their knowledge, understanding, skills and competence to deliver the clinical governance agenda at a local or individual level. Local support for staff could be in the form of:

- *Clinical supervision*: offering a framework for staff to identify and explore issues about the quality of care delivered, along with the

Internal	External
Financial • Funding for staff support and equipment, e.g. clinical audit, personnel etc. • Back fill costs for staff attending courses • The development of courses	**Locally** • Collaboration with other healthcare agencies and patient/carers support groups • Developing partnerships with universities, education establishments
Resources • Education • Supervision • Time out • Access to information • Expert and practical advice • Accommodation • Equipment • Support from management • Trust board commitment	**Nationally** • Links to the: – Department of Health – Healthcare Commission – NICE – Professional regulatory bodies – National Patient Safety Agency – Clinical Governance Support Team

Fig. 5.3 Internal and external factors supporting clinical governance.

identification of education and training needs in enabling them to improve their clinical competence.
- *Reflective practice and critical incident analysis*: to help identify and resolve clinical concerns and share good practice.
- *Lifelong learning*: the need to ensure that staff have the support to continuously develop professionally.
- *Performance management review*: to offer support and advice in the organisation's drive for continuous quality improvement.
- *Clinical audit*: to support staff in the evaluation of care associated with set standards and guidelines.
- *Offering the opportunity for networking and collaboration*: to encourage staff to share and learn from each other.
- *Professional self-regulation*: offering support and encouragement for the development of the professions' and individuals' performances as outlined by the National Clinical Assessment Authority.

National support comes in the form of:

- *National Institute for Clinical Excellence*: by setting clear national standards to provide clear guidance to the NHS on clinical and cost effectiveness across a wide range of health interventions, and the development of services.
- *National service frameworks*: directed at raising national standards of care and reducing unacceptable variations in care provision, e.g. coronary heart disease, mental health.
- *Care Quality Commission:* to provide support by independently reviewing local efforts to improve the quality of health care by the implementation of the clinical governance systems and processes.DH (2001b)
- *National patient Safety Agency:* designed to support a develop learning from patient safety incidents.
- *National Health Service Litigation Authority:* provides information and standards (CNST) on risk patient, legal advice and claims handling.
- *National Institute for Mental Health:* Provides advice, guidance and best available evidence for mental health practice.
- *National Clinical Governance Support Team:* provides expert advice and a series of development programmes for NHS boards and clinical teams.

Without the correct and adequate local and national support for staff, to assist with their endeavours at an organisation, team and individual level to introduce clinical governance, the implementation and evaluation of clinical governance will not happen. Perhaps this accounts for the government's section in the National Plan in 2000 about the 'NHS will support and value its staff' (DH 2000, p. 4), directed towards resolving the fundamental barriers associated with the provision of support.

> **Activity 5.1 Feedback: establishing the barriers to implementing clinical governance.**
>
> The barriers associated with the implementation of clinical governance can be classified into seven themes:
>
> - Culture
> - Management
> - Leadership
> - Communication
> - Education and training
> - Knowledge
> - Support

By exploring these barriers, which tend to be viewed negatively, it is possible to develop positive strategies for the successful implementation of clinical governance systems and processes at an organisation, team and individual level.

Conclusion

This chapter shows how the implementation of clinical governance depends on resolving the potential barriers that exist within the organisation, teams and individuals – barriers which, if left unresolved, will make the linking of the systems and processes associated with the implementation of clinical governance difficult to achieve. These barriers can be classified into key themes associated with culture, management, leadership, communication, education and training, knowledge and support. As individual healthcare professionals, it is imperative that we understand the existence of these barriers and develop strategies to overcome them. Failure to embrace this challenge will make clinical governance difficult to implement in our daily practices.

Key points

The barriers to clinical governance:

- Refer to an obstruction or blockage in one or several of the complex systems and processes that make up clinical governance
- Can be classified as internal and external factors attributed to individuals or organisations

- Can be themed into seven key headings for which strategies require development in resolving their impact at an organisation, team and individual level: culture, management, leadership, communication, education and training, knowledge, and support
- Management, leadership styles and culture are three barriers which cannot be overlooked from either an organisation, team or individual level when considering the implementation of clinical governance
- A closer inspection of these barriers will offer positive and constructive ways of achieving clinical governance
- Adequate support is necessary
- Education and training for staff on clinical governance is essential.

Suggested reading

Department of Health (2001) *Assuring the Quality of Medical Practice: Implementing Supporting Doctors Protecting Patients*. DH, London.

Stewart, R. (1996) *Leading in the NHS: A Practical Guide*, 2nd edn. Macmillan Business, London.

References

Allen A. (1993) Changing theory in nursing practice. *Senior Nurse*, 13 (1) 43–44.

Care Quality Commission (2009) *Guidance for Healthcare Professionals*. CQC, London, http://www.cqc.org.uk/guidanceforprofessionals/healthcare.cfm. Accessed 18 November 2009.

Collins, W. (1987) *Collins Universal English Dictionary*. Readers Union Ltd, Glasgow.

Cullen, R., Nichols, S. & Halligan, A. (2000) NHS support team. Reviewing a service – discovering the unwritten rules. *British Journal of Clinical Governance*, 5 (4) 233–239.

Davies, H.T.O., Nutley, S.M. & Mannion, R. (2000) Organizational culture and quality of health care. *Quality in Health Care*, 9, 111–119.

Department of Health (2000) *National Plan*. DH, London.

Department of Health (2001a) *Interim Guidance on Post-Mortem Examinations*. 5 January. http:/www.doh.gov.uk/postmortem.htm.

Department of Health (2001b) *Assuring the Quality of Medical Practice: Implementing Supporting Doctors Protecting Patients*. Department of Health, London.

Department of Health (2004a) *Committee of Inquiry to Investigate How the NHS Handled Allegations About the Performance and Conduct of Richard Neale*. DH, London.

Department of Health (2004b) *Standards for Better Health: Health Care Standards for Services Under the NHS/ A Consultation Document*. DH, London.

DTI (1997) *Partnership with People*. Department of Trade and Industry, London.

Edwards, J. & Packham, R. (1999) A model for the practical implementation of clinical governance. *Journal of Clinical Excellence*, 1 (1) 13–18.

Harvey, G. (1998) Improving patient care. *RCN Magazine*, Autumn, 8–9.
Haslock, I. (1999) Introducing clinical governance in an acute trust. *Hospital Medicine*, 60 (10) 745–747.
Hawkins, S. & Shohet, R. (1989) *Supervision in the Helping Professions*. Open University Press, Milton Keynes.
Kotter, J.P. & Schlesinger, L.A. (1979) Choosing strategies for change. *Harvard Business Review*, 57 (2) 106–115.
Lancaster, J. & Lancaster, W. (1982) *The Nurse as the Change Agent*. Mosby, St Louis.
MacDonald, A. (1996) Responding to the results of the Beverly Allitt inquiry. *Nursing Times*, 92 (2) 23–25.
Marquis, B. L. & Hutson, C. J. (2000) *Leadership Roles and Management Function in NHS Institute for Innovation and Improvement* (2009) http://www.institute.nhs.uk/. Accessed 18 November 2009.
McSherry, R. (1999) Supporting patients and their families. In: *Caring for the Seriously Ill Patient* (eds C.C. Bassett & L. Mahin). Arnold, London.
McSherry, R. & Simmons, M. (2001) The importance of research dissemination and the barriers to implementation. In: *Evidence-Informed Nursing: A Guide for Clinical Nurses* (eds R. McSherry, M. Simmons & P. Abbott). Routledge, London.
McSherry, R., Simmons, M. & Abbott, P. (2001) *Evidence-Informed Nursing: A Guide for Clinical Nurses*. Routledge, London.
Manley, K (2005) Transformational culture: a culture of effectiveness. Cited in McCormack, B, Manley, K, Garbett, R (eds) Practice Development in Nursing Blackwell Publishing, Oxford.
Mullally, S (2001) Leadership and politics Nursing Management 8, 4, 21–27.
NHS Leadership Centre (2002) *NHS Leadership Qualities Framework* http://www.nhsleadershipqualities.nhs.uk. Accessed 18 November 2009.
Marquis, B. L. & Hutson, C. J. (2000) *Nursing: Theory and Application*, 3rd edn. Lippincott, Philadelphia, USA.
Northcott, N. (1999) Organizational effectiveness. *Nursing Times Learning Curve*, 3 (1) 10.
O'Neill, S. (2000) Clinical governance in action Part 4: Communication. *Professional Nurse*, 16 (1) 816–817.
Parker, D. & Hudson, P. (2001) Understanding your culture. Shell International Exploration and production, Rijswijk.
Potter, A.P. & Perry G.A. (1993) *Foundations of Nursing: Concepts, Process and Practice*. Mosby, London.
Ramsey, S. (2001) Audit exposes UK's worst serial killer. *The Lancet*, 357, 13 January, 123–124.
Slim (1996) *Cited in Leading In The NHS: A Practical Guide*, 2nd edn. (ed. R. Stewart). Macmillan Business, London.
Stewart, R. (1996) *Leading In The NHS: A Practical Guide*, 2nd edn. Macmillan Business, London.
The Lancet (1998) Editorial. First lessons from the 'Bristol case'. *The Lancet*, 351 (117), 1669.
Westrum, R. (1992) Cultures with requisite imagination. In: Verification and Validation of Complex Systems: Human Factors Issues (eds J. Wise, O. Hopkin & P. Stager). Springer, Berlin, pp. 401–416.

Chapter 6

Clinical Governance and the Law

John Tingle

Introduction: defining terms

In focusing a legal discussion, lawyers are always keen to seek definitions of terms and to identify the parameters of discussion. Definitions and identification of parameters bring clarity and certainty. Clients can be advised where they stand and can organise their affairs accordingly. Can this lawyer's exercise be usefully attempted with the term clinical governance? Is there one absolute definition that everyone subscribes to without exception and are there identifiable parameters to the topic?

On reading this book, a number of definitions of the term do seem possible and the parameters of the topic do appear unclear. A lot can be seen to come under the term. In view of this fluidity of nature, it would seem appropriate to view clinical governance as one of those umbrella-type terms, like accountability, patient empowerment or lifelong learning. With these terms the focus is less on the term or label itself, but more on the ideas behind them. When the ideas behind the label are looked at, commonalities can often be seen to emerge.

We now have the term 'integrated governance'; clinical governance would appear to be a component element of this umbrella coordinating principle. The DH (2006) state:

> 'Integrated Governance' is a co-ordinating principle. It does not seek to replace or supersede clinical or financial governance-or any other governance domain. Rather re-energises their vital importance and the inter-dependence and inter-connection between them.

From the perspective of the individual healthcarer, clinical governance would seem essentially to be about doing your job well and helping to ensure the delivery of good quality, safe healthcare and services. Legal topics relevant to clinical governance could therefore range from health and safety law, employment law, ethical issues and dilemmas in medicine and nursing law, to consent, negligence, complaints, patient rights, and so on. In fact the legal discussion could be almost endless because of the fluid nature of the concept and the wide range of topics that can be encompassed within the term.

In order to provide a reasoned legal treatment of relevant concepts the discussion in this chapter will be focused on clinical negligence. This area seems to best illustrate the relationship between clinical governance and the law.

Litigation in the NHS: caring in a rights-based culture

Clinical negligence and complaints about healthcare have shown an upward trend over the years, it is beyond doubt that patients are now much more informed about their rights and that they live in a rights-based culture. Alleged infringements of Human Rights are regularly featured in the media and are hot political topics. The NHS Constitution (DH 2009) clearly articulates a rights-based NHS culture:

> As well as capturing the purpose, principles and values of the NHS, the Constitution brings together a number of rights, pledges and responsibilities for staff and patients alike. These rights and responsibilities are the result of extensive discussions and consultations with staff, patients and public and it reflects what matters to them.

It is clear that the concept of clinical governance is now being applied at a very difficult time in the NHS's history. The NHS is in an almost constant state of reform and flux and the demand for finite NHS resources seems almost infinite. Everybody is demanding more from the NHS and patient expectations seem set at a very high level. It is perhaps worth reflecting on whether patient's expectations might have been set at too higher level by successive Governments and healthcarers with initiatives such as the Patient's Charter and now the NHS Constitution. Given the complexity of modern medicine, the dependence on the human element, professional skills and judgments; surely risk, errors and adverse incidents are going to be an inevitable feature of any healthcare system? We can try our best at managing them through good clinical risk management and patient safety strategies but they can never all be totally eliminated. We may perhaps have given our patients a too rosy view of what can actually be achieved in a socialised healthcare structure such as the NHS?

There is however no room for complacency, the NHS is a high-risk enterprise; the Healthcare Commission gave some figures on patient safety (Healthcare Commission 2009a):

> Various studies have been conducted, in the UK and internationally, in an attempt to discover the level of harm done to patients as a consequence of receiving healthcare services. Estimates range from less than 3% to over 16% of patients experiencing an 'adverse event', with around 50% of these being preventable and around 20% being life threatening or fatal. While healthcare, by its very nature, incurs some inherent risk, such levels of harm are unacceptable and the boards of NHS trusts cannot afford to overlook such glaring statistics.
>
> The NHS does not presently manifest an ingrained patient safety culture; progress in developing one nationally is patchy.

To sue or not to sue

When a patient is injured by the NHS a complaint or even litigation may follow but not always. The National Health Service Litigation Authority (NHSLA) annual report states (NHSLA 2009a):

> 2008/09 saw a significant increase in the number of claims received, compared with the same period last year. Clinical claims rose by more than 11% and non-clinical claims by over 10%. The preceding five years had seen a largely static intake of new claims and we have not been able to identify any single factor that might have precipitated the rise.

On outstanding liabilities the NHSLA state: (NHSLA 2009b);

> As at 31 March 2009, the NHSLA estimates that it has potential liabilities of £13.51 billion, of which £13.37 billion relate to clinical negligence claims (the remainder being liabilities under PES and LTPS). This figure represents the estimated value of all known claims, together with an actuarial estimate of those incurred but not yet reported (IBNR), which may settle or be withdrawn over future years.

The Healthcare Commission (HC 2009b) state that NHS organisations receive about 135 000 complaints annually, noting that:

> In an organisation the size of the NHS, which provides over 380 million treatments each year, this is, overall, a very small percentage.

They go on to express some concern that patients and the public do not always complain when they do receive poor or even unsafe service, The Healthcare Commission HC (2009b):

> However, we remain concerned that patients and the public do not always complain when they do receive poor or even unsafe service. It is vital that patients feel that they can complain to NHS organisations without prejudicing the healthcare they receive.

In a very real sense complaints can be good for an organisation as they show 'real-time' was is happening in their area and how the service can be improved. Properly handled a complaint can be a jewel; it can provide a valuable insight into organisational health. The gold standard would be to term every complainant into an advocate for the organisation complained against.

How the courts determine competent clinical practice

Competent clinical practice is a basic and essential prerequisite for the effective delivery of clinical governance. As a matter of common sense, if you practise safely and reflectively the risks of adverse incidents will be reduced and quality clinical practices will be maintained.

Almost every day stories appear in the press about medical mishaps with patients being injured. The notable medical scandals of Shipman, Alder Hay and Bristol have certainly focused the public's attention. A mishap however is not necessarily negligence, sometimes accidents just happen and nobody is at fault. For an accident or mishap to sound in the award of compensation, the tort of negligence must be committed. The burden of proving negligence lies on the claimant patient and there are quite a number of high legal hurdles to overcome. It should however be stated at the outset that most cases clinical negligence cases do not proceed to court. The NHSLA (NHSLA 2009a) state on the outcome of claims:

> Whenever possible and appropriate, we attempt to settle claims without litigation. Of the 8885 clinical and non-clinical claims where a formal letter of claim was received in 2008/09, typically less than 4% will go to Court. The historical figure of 4% does not include claims settled by individual NHS organisations within their excess and open incidents investigated but not yet proceeded with as a claim.

In order to succeed in a malpractice action, the claimant or plaintiff (these words mean the same thing) must show that a legal duty of care existed towards the patient that the duty was broken and that legally recognised damage was caused. For the purposes of this discussion the focus will be on the breach of duty.

A patient may complain, for example, that pressure sores were allowed to develop and were then not treated properly. There was no initial pressure sore risk assessment done and the sores just got worse. The patient has been off work for a number of weeks and this, they argue, could have been prevented had the nurse systematically assessed them for pressure sores and then treated them properly. The nurse, the patient argues, is in breach of their legal duty of care by not systematically assessing them, and then failing to treat the sores that developed. The nurse has behaved improperly and malpractice has occurred.

The word properly is important here. What is meant by this term? Lawyers would not necessarily know what proper treatment would be; they are not doctors or nurses, though some could well be. They would ask for an expert report from a leading wound care specialist and ask them, not what they would have done, but what they would have expected the ordinary skilled nurse in the relevant specialty to have done in the circumstances of the case. They need to determine the standard of care. The courts would not necessarily expect best practice but reasonable practice, though this is an issue of legal debate and conjecture. Legally, competent, proper clinical practice is reasonable practice determined by reference to the famous Bolam case.

Lord Browne-Wilkinson in *Bolitho v. City and Hackney HA* [1998] Lloyds Rep Med 26 (p. 31) said this on the standard of care and referred to Bolam:

> The locus classicus of the test for the standard of care required of a doctor or any other person professing some skill or competence is the direction to the jury given by McNair J in Bolam v. Friern Hospital Management Committee [1957] 1 WLR 583, 587:
>
> I myself would prefer to put it this way, that he is not guilty of negligence if he has acted in accordance with a practice accepted as proper by a responsible body of medical men skilled in that particular art ... Putting it the other way round, a man is not negligent, if he is acting in accordance with such a practice, merely because there is a body of opinion who would take a contrary view.

Over the years the courts have been seen to be reluctant to challenge what experts have said about reasonable medical practices when assessing the standard of care, being unduly deferential to doctors, a theme made clear by Britain's most senior judge, the Lord Chief Justice, Lord Woolf (*The Times* 2001):

> . . . until recently the courts treated the medical profession with excessive deference, but recently the position has changed . . . The over deferential approach is captured by the phrase 'Doctor knows best'. The contemporary approach is a more critical approach. It could be said to be that Doctor knows best if he acts reasonably and logically and gets his facts right.

The courts can be seen to have adopted a more proactive approach to testing medical evidence and determining the standard of care. The Bolitho case is the baseline case for the new approach.

The case involved a 2-year-old plaintiff who was re-admitted to hospital on 16 January 1984 after suffering a serious bout of the croup. On 17 January his condition deteriorated and there were two occasions where he had episodes of acute breathing problems. Twice the nurse observing him summoned the paediatric registrar but there was no response to the calls. The plaintiff suffered a third episode, which led to cardiac arrest and severe anoxic brain damage. It was accepted for the defendant that the failure of doctors to attend amounted to a breach of the duty of care. However it was claimed that had they attended they would not have intubated.

> Although this was a defence based essentially on lack of causation . . . to succeed it required the court to accept that the hypothetical failure to intubate in such a case would not itself have been a breach of duty. In this regard, the defendant adduced evidence from a number of expert witnesses to the effect that faced with a patient exhibiting the plaintiff's history and symptoms, they too would not intubate . . . The House of Lords agreed, held that the hypothetical decision not to intubate the plaintiff would have been in accord with responsible medical practice. (Stauch *et al.* 2006)

The plaintiff lost his case. Lord Browne-Wilkinson stated the following:

> . . . [I]n my view, the court is not bound to hold that a defendant doctor escapes liability for negligent treatment or diagnosis just because he leads evidence from a number of medical experts who are genuinely of opinion that the defendant's treatment or diagnosis accorded with sound medical practice . . . The use of these adjectives responsible, reasonable and respectable all show that the court has to be satisfied that the exponents of the body of opinion relied upon can demonstrate that such opinion has a logical basis. In particular in cases involving, as they so often do, the weighing of risks against benefits, the judge before accepting a body of opinion as being responsible, reasonable, or respectable, will need to be satisfied that, in forming their views, the

> experts have directed their minds to the question of comparative risks and benefits and have reached a defensible conclusion on the matter. (p. 302, Stauch *et al.* 2006)

The Bolitho case reconsidered the Bolam test and placed it within context. Bolam has been returned to its proper limits and appropriate context, as Brazier and Miola (2000) conclude on the Bolitho decision:

> The decision does, however signal judicial will, at the highest level, to return Bolam to its proper context. Together with the many other factors prompting change, inappropriate deference to medical opinion should be replaced by legal principles which recognise the imperative to listen to both doctors and patients and which acknowledge that the medical professional is just as much required to justify his or her practice as the architect or solicitor.

The court's contemporary approach to determining the standard of care in medical malpractice can be regarded as evidence-based approach, which fits in well with clinical governance. Foster (1998) feels that evidence-based medicine might begin to play a part in malpractice litigation after the Bolitho case:

> If the published evidence makes a wholly one-sided case against a particular medical practice, it will be difficult for any expert to say that its adoption by the defendant was reasonable, even though he or she is in august medical company in doing so.

The law and clinical guidelines

Judges today will now be more influenced by national and local clinical guidelines issued by hospitals, NICE, the Royal Medical Colleges and other bodies that produce guidelines. This can be seen in the case of *Penney, Palmer and Cannon v. East Kent Health Authority* [2000] Lloyds Rep Med 41, discussed by Tingle and Rodgers (1999). This case concerned cervical smear tests and negligence allegations concerning interpretation of findings. Some slides had been labelled negatively when they should not have been and there was no medical follow-up for the claimants who subsequently went on to develop invasive adenocarcinoma of the cervix and had to undergo surgery, which included a hysterectomy. The Court of Appeal held, dismissing the Health Authority's appeal, that because of the observable abnormalities on the slides they should not have been labelled negative. The standards of the CSP (cervical screening programme) were not complied with and consequently the Health

Authority was liable in negligence. The trial judge had relied on a test of screener satisfaction known as 'the absolute confidence test', which according to the judge all the experts seemed to endorse. The trial judge had used this test in deciding the issue of the correct standard of care and whether this standard had been met. This test is incorporated into the clinical guidelines of the CSP.

This case shows clinical guidelines influencing judges and is a theme which should continue as NICE issues more guidelines.

The practice of evidence-based healthcare based on clinical guidelines is one way of demonstrating effective clinical governance. The courts would seem to support and use this approach in assessing whether malpractice has taken place or not. It could well be argued that reasonable clinical practice is no longer the acceptable judicial benchmark of appropriateness of clinical conduct. If most healthcarers are practising evidence-based best clinical practice, then surely the standard shifts from reasonable to best practice? In time cases will clarify this point.

Personal updating: knowledge and clinical guidelines

Professional staff development is an important aspect to demonstrating clinical governance and is the hallmark of a professional person. We would all expect professionals to keep up to date with changes and developments in their field of expertise. We rely on them and do not have the skill to second-guess them. In the healthcare context the expectations of professional updating are no different. It is possible that a malpractice case could be brought by a patient who argues that the doctor or nurse was negligent in not applying an appropriate clinical guideline which would have helped them make a full recovery, or even some widely available research. A case could proceed on the basis of negligence through ignorance. A court would take the view that the reasonable doctor or nurse would be expected to keep up with professional developments in their sphere of practice, but what does this really entail? A doctor or nurse may read one article in the professional press about treating one condition and another may come out the following week advocating a different course of treatment. It is often said that medicine is not a science but a scientific-based art.

According to the present state of the law, minority medical or nursing opinion can still be Bolam reasonable with the caveat that the court will test the views. The courts will look for a logical basis and a risk benefit analysis. Clinical guidelines, nationally endorsed, may assist the court but would not be determinative. Each case will often depend on its own facts. Clinical guidelines do not suspend clinical autonomy. There is often more than one reasonable and logical way to care for a patient. A patient's condition may also contraindicate the application of the guideline or treatment. The healthcarer should always be prepared to advance a reasonable reason for not following the guideline or the usual course of treatment. Two cases assist on this issue.

In the case of *Crawford v. Board of Governors of Charing Cross Hospital* (*The Times*, 8 December 1953) the plaintiff developed brachial palsy as a result of his arm being kept in an extended position, at an angle of 808 from the body position, during an operation. Six months before an article had appeared in *The Lancet* pointing out this danger. The anaesthetist had not read the article in question and the judge at first instance, Gerrard J., held the defendants liable for negligence. The Court of Appeal allowed the hospital's appeal and found the anaesthetist not negligent. Lord Denning stated that:

> it would, I think, be putting too high a burden on a medical man to say that he has to read every article appearing in the current medical press; and it would be quite wrong to suggest that a medical man is negligent because he does not at once put into operation the suggestions which some contributor or other might make in a medical journal. The time may come in a particular case when a new recommendation may be so well proved and so well known, and so well accepted that it should be adopted, but that was not so in this case. (Mason & McCall Smith 1999)

Mason and McCall Smith (1999) comment:

> Failure to read a single article, it was said, may be excusable, while disregard of a series of warnings in the medical press could well be evidence of negligence. In view of the rapid progress currently being made in many areas of medicine, and in view of the amount of information confronting the average doctor, it is unreasonable to expect a doctor to be aware of every development in his field. At the same time, he must be reasonably up to date and must know of major developments ... The practice of medicine has, however, become increasingly based on principles of scientific elucidation and report and the pressure on doctors to keep abreast of current developments is now considerable. It is no longer possible for a doctor to coast along on the basis of long experience; such an attitude has been firmly discredited not only in medicine but in many other professions and callings.

The views expressed by the authors are the attitude that courts would take today. Crawford was a case in 1953; the information technology age is now firmly with us.

A more contemporary case on staff updating is *Gascoine v. Ian Sheridan and Co and Latham* [1994] 5 Med LR 437. This case concerned a number of issues, one of which was the responsibility of a consultant to keep informed about changes and developments in his specialty. Mitchell J. said that the consultant in the case was a very busy man 'who clearly had a responsibility to keep himself generally informed on mainstream changes in diagnosis treatment and practice through the mainstream literature such as the leading textbooks and *The Journal of Obstetrics and Gynaecology*'. The judge went on to say that it would be unreasonable for the consultant to 'acquaint himself with the content of the more obscure journals'.

A balance has to be drawn. The healthcarer should, at the very least, be prepared to demonstrate a systematic updating regime; just saying that you do not have the time to keep up to date is not enough. An awareness of the main clinical guidelines in the relevant specialty should also be demonstrated.

Good guidelines practice

We have seen that clinical guidelines can be used to convey evidence-based practice. Effective evidence-based practice demonstrates clinical governance in action.

It is always good common-sense practice to date and sign a clinical guideline, and say who was involved in drafting it and what evidence was used. Always build in review dates. If you do not, how can you say that best practice is being followed? Practice changes, so a guideline should be reviewed. It is also worth stating on the guideline that the user must always use their own clinical judgement and that the guideline does not suspend this. These are common-sense steps, as guidelines could conceivably become the subject of legal actions. A patient could argue that a guideline was negligently designed and they have suffered as a result, or that another guideline should have been used. We have seen in the Penney case above how courts can treat guidelines. The DH also produces useful advice on using clinical guidelines (DoH 1996) and identifies a number of legal considerations:

'(1) the objectives for the clinical guidelines need to be clear, and clearly stated. This will affect their subsequent legal standing;
(2) the intended use and applicability of clinical guidelines should be spelt out clearly, in the introduction;
(3) the guidelines must make clear for whom they are intended. The recommendations will usually be intended for a particular group of practitioners;

(4) clinical guidelines that no longer reflect best practice might conceivably become actionable, and developers need to incorporate specific statements about their validity and review procedure;
(5) they should be constructed in such a way that allows deviation and does not suffocate initiative that might bring about further improvements;
(6) the development of clinical guidelines must involve all the relevant professions and managers.'

This booklet provides lots of common-sense advice and should be read in conjunction with the advice offered on the NICE website: http://www.nice.org.uk/niceMedia/pdf/Legal_context_nice_guidance.pdf.

Guideline developers need to create in essence an audit trail of their work as the information will prove useful in defending any claim of malpractice.

In conclusion, the law can be seen as an important mechanism to advance clinical governance. The courts are sensitive to the issues of evidence-based practice and the need to test clinical practice. Judges are not as deferential as they once were. Litigation and complaints are on the increase but the government can be seen to be developing key strategies to instil more confidence in the NHS. More, however, can be done at the NHS workface to develop an engrained patient safety culture. All clinical staff and their management need to take patient safety more seriously. Clinical governance is just one tool being used and there are a number of others. Professionals have a legal duty to keep up to date and cases have gone to court on this area. Clinical guidelines are an important quality development tool and a way of demonstrating the existence of the practice of evidence-based care and the operation of clinical governance. The courts remain the final arbiters of what is acceptable clinical practice and they are the ultimate and final mechanism of clinical accountability.

References

Brazier, M. & Miola, J. (2000) Bye-bye Bolam: a medical litigation revolution? *Medical Law Review*, 8 (1) Spring, 85–114.

Department of Health (2006) *Integrated Governance Handbook*. February 2006. Department of Health, London.

Department of Health (2009) *The NHS Constitution*. http://www.dh.gov.uk/en/Healthcare/NHSConstitution/index.htm. Accessed 29th September 2009.

Department of Health (1996) *Clinical Guidelines, Using Clinical Guidelines to Improve Patient Care within the NHS*. Department of Health, London.

Foster, C. (1998) Bolam: consolidation and clarification. *Health Care Risk Report*, 4 (5) April, 5–7.
Healthcare Commission (2009a) *Safe in the Knowledge*, March. Healthcare Commission, London.
Healthcare Commission (2009b) *Spotlight on Complaints*, February. Healthcare Commission, London.
Mason, J.K. & McCall Smith, R.A. (1999) *Law and Medical Ethics*, 5th edn. Butterworths, London.
NHSLA (2009a) *The National Health Service Litigation Authority*. Annual Report and Accounts 2009. TSO, London.
NHSLA (2009b) The NHS Litigation Authority, Factsheet 2: financial information. Accessed 29th September 2009. http://www.nhsla.com/NR/rdonlyres/465D7ABD-239F-4273-A01E-C0CED557453D/0/NHSLAFactsheet2financialinformation200809.doc.
Stauch, M. & Wheat, K. with Tingle, J.H. (2006) *Text, Cases and Materials on Medical Law*, 3rd edn. Routledge-Cavendish, Abingdon, Oxon.
The Times (2001) On-line Wednesday 17 January 2001, Lord Woolf's speech in full. Accessed 18th January 2001. http://www.thetimes.co.uk/article/0.2-69685.00.html.
Tingle, J.H. & Rodgers, M.E. (1999) Clinical guidelines, NICE and the court of appeal. *Nottingham Law School Journal*, 8 (2), 172.

Chapter 7

The Impact of Clinical Governance in the National Health Service

Rob McSherry and Paddy Pearce

Introduction

The chapter will explore the empirical and contemporary literature to demonstrate the impact of clinical governance at an individual, team and organisational level. The relative merits and demerits of clinical governance will be debated.

Clinical governance friend or foe?

When clinical governance was introduced into the NHS in 1997 (DH 1997) there was a degree of cynicism about its ability to achieve its goals because healthcare professionals were divided in their opinions. 'The subject is one which divides doctors [indeed all healthcare professionals] into two groups. The minority believe that clinical governance will prove to be a useful tool for introducing quality improvements into health care, whereas the majority consists of those cynics who believe the topic is another "flavour of the month" which will go away if ignored' (Gaminiara 2000 p. 80). Dependent on your viewpoint clinical governance was either embraced or resisted. Whilst acknowledging the range of views from the cynics to the optimists, clinical governance as unfortunately or fortunately began to be accepted as part of the NHS culture of today. As Halligan (2006) suggests clinical governance is hear to stay. 'The brand with its implicit promise of patient-centred, accountable care has put down roots into healthcare culture. Despite the initial perceptions of threat and challenge to organisational and clinical autonomy sometimes flagged up by

Clinical Governance, third edition. By Rob McSherry and Paddy Pearce.
Published 2011 by Blackwell Publishing Ltd.

the phrase, it has become part of the vernacular of the NHS' (p. 6). Whilst agreeing with Halligan's (2006) view, we would suggest this need to be substantiated with the backing of empirical evidence. The notion of demonstrating the impact of clinical governance is imperative given the fact that its principles have transcended into almost all healthcare disciplines; for instance, dentistry, pharmacy, prison healthcare services, Primary Care Trusts, Independent Sector to name but a few. The concept seems to have permeated from the hierarchy of boards to the grass roots where clinical practice occurs. However, what evidence is available to justify its relative merits and demerits to individuals, teams and organisations.

A literature search on Goggle highlighted over 1.6 million hits associated with clinical governance demonstrating its popularity across the globe. Similarly the various healthcare databases like CINHAL and MEDLINE reveal a proliferation of literature defining the key components and associated issues of clinical governance within the healthcare setting. However a critical review and synthesis of this literature illustrates minimal empirical-based studies demonstrating the impact of clinical governance.

Revealing the impact of clinical governance

The impact of clinical governance is emerging through the undertaking of empirical-based evaluation studies. We have found relatively few robust well-designed studies that seek to evaluate the impact of clinical governance

However, we would like to acknowledge that this is not a systematic review or indeed an in-depth critical review of all the empirical studies available. It is our intention to raise awareness of the importance of focusing on evaluating the impact of clinical governance. We believe this is imperative given the significant amount of finances and resource invested in implementing clinical governance which according to National Audit Office (NAO) was estimated to cost the NHS approximately £60 million in 2002–2003 (NAO 2003, p. 4). A critical review of six studies by (Hartley *et al.* 2002; Degeling *et al.* 2003; NAO 2003; Freeman & Walshe 2004; Wallace *et al.* 2004) and Braithwaite & Travaglia (Table 7.1) provides some evidence to demonstrate the impact of clinical governance at national and regional level. It is evident that clinical governance is making a difference in the following five key areas: accountability, organisational structures, continuous quality improvement, performance management and culture. The reminder of this section will focus on highlighting how clinical governance has influenced these areas both positively and negatively.

Table 7.1 Research studies reporting on the impact pf clinical governance (in chronological order).

Author (s) and year: Braithwaite & Travaglia (2008)
Origin: Australia
Title: An overview of clinical governance policies, practices and initiatives
Purpose: To map and define clinical governance and explore the implications for Boards and Executives wishing to promote clinical governance
Method: Systematic literature including grey material
Sample: Medline and CINAHL searched 1996–2006
Main findings:

- Links are made between health services clinical and corporate governance
- The use of clinical governance in the promotion of patient safety
- A focus on quality assurance and continuous improvement
- Acknowledges that clinical governance is relatively new and is increasingly accepted as an approach to quality improvement and patient safety
- Concludes that all stakeholders need to be involved
- Boards involvement is vital

Author (s) and year: Freeman & Walshe (2004)
Origin: England
Title: Achieving progress through clinical governance, a national study of healthcare managers perception in the NHS in England
Purpose: To explore the perception of progress made with Clinical Governance
Method: Quantitative method using the Organisational Progress in Clinical Governance (OPCG) schedule
Sample: Random sample ($n = 100$) Board members and directorate managers of English acute, mental health/learning difficulties trusts.
Main findings:

- Evidence that structures for Clinical Governance are established
- More progress has been made with assurance and corporate accountability
- Progress is less advanced in quality improvement, leadership and collaborative working
- Managers perceptions of achievement were slightly lower that those of Board members

Table 7.1 (*cont'd*)

Author (s) and year: Wallace, Boxall & Spurgeon (2004)
Origin: England
Title: Organisational change through clinician governance: the West Midlands 3 years on
Purpose: To examine the perception of clinical governance leads 2.5 years after a baseline assessment.
Method: Survey-using semi-structured telephone interviews
Sample: All 40 NHS Trusts in the West Midlands, England, UK
Main findings:

- Expected outcomes were achieved more often than expected than at the time of the baseline assessment.
- Improved patient outcomes and documented changes in clinical behaviour were expected and achieved
- A more open culture was evident in 84% of Trusts
- A new approach to consultant appraisal and critical incidents was welcomed
- League tables and external review had an adverse effects were results were poor, however where results were positive the impact was small.

Author (s) and year: Degeling, Maxwell, Coyle & MacBeth (2003)
Origin: Wales
Title: The impact of CHI: evidence from Wales
Purpose:
Method: Survey and Focus groups from
Sample: Six welsh Trusts
Main findings:

- CHI's Clinical Governance Reviews seems to have had little impact on the NHS
- For CHI to be more effective they need to more away from assessing the seven pillars of clinical governance
- Healthcare professional have different experiences with understanding evaluations of clinical governance
- Each professional group seems to be influenced by its professional culture
- CHI needs to increase its awareness of how grass roots clinical staff perceive and evaluate clinical governance
- CHI need to provide a very clear message about the specific changes in practice and culture is seeking to achieve.

Table 7.1 (*cont'd*)

Author (s) and year: National Audit Office (2003)
Origin: England
Title: Achieving improvement through clinical governance: a progress report on implementation by NHS Trusts
Purpose: To provide the UK government with an independent assessment of progress made with the implementation of clinical governance
Method:

- A Census of NHS Trust
- Survey of Board members and Senior Managers
- Review of reports from CHI
- Interviews with DH and regional staff

Sample: A combined total of 100 Acute NHS Trusts, Mental Health Trusts and Ambulance Trusts
Main findings:

- Implementation of clinical governance has raised the profile quality issues for boards of NHS Trust
- Virtually all NHS Trusts have laid the necessary foundations, but not all of the components of clinical governance are fully embedded in all clinical directorates
- The implementation of clinical governance between and within Trust is patchy
- There is greater accountability for clinical performance in Trusts
- There has been a change in clinical culture becoming more transparent
- There is evidence of more collaborative working
- Evidence of improvements in practice and patient care, yet Trust still require robust process for measuring overall progress
- There remain room for improvement with:
  - The provision of support for the implementation of clinical governance
  - Communication between NHS Boards and clinical directorates
  - The development of a coherent approach: to quality improvement, processes for risk management and performance management and the systematic dissemination of sharing lessons learnt with the rest of the NHS
- Where NHS Trusts have been more successful with the implementation of clinical governance. The key features identified were:
  - Strong leadership
  - Commitment to staff
  - Willingness to consider doing things differently

Table 7.1 (*cont'd*)

Author (s) and year: Hartley, Griffiths, Saunders (2002) **Origin:** England **Title:** An evaluation of clinical governance in the public health departments of the West Midlands Region to assess two models for examining clinical governance in public health- namely the model produced by Faculty of Public Health and the West Midlands SPOCK model **Purpose:** To evaluate the development of clinical governance in public health department **Method:** Semi-structured interviews carried out during the annual visit by the regional director of public health **Sample:** All Health Authorities in West Midlands region. Directors of public health **Main findings:** • Both models were useful in examining clinical governance • A combination of both model produced better results • West Midlands public health department value annual visits as they provided external peer review • Public health departments have ownership of the process • Most departments felt that clinical governance provided a framework to bring together a range existing governance activities into a more coherent whole • Appraisal and CPD were well addressed • Half of the departments report good resource allocation for clinical governance • Nine departments felt that clinical governance had a high organisational profile

Accountability

Freeman and Walshe's (2004) study reported that clinical governance has played a major role in highlighting and improving corporate accountability structures with NHS Trusts. Corporate accountability in this instance referred to the efficiency and effectiveness of NHS Boards, Committees and associated systems and processes for managing and dealing with clinical risks or quality related issues. Whilst it is evident that significant progress has been made in changing attitudes at Executive and Board levels, Freeman and Walshe's (2004) study revealed a difference in the perception of progress between managers and directors. Similarly the NAO (2003) study concluded that clinical governance has raised the profile of quality issues for corporate boards, yet there remains a degree of inconsistency between and within the various NHS organisations. Hartley *et al.*

(2002) study provides some insight of the impact of clinical governance relating to the importance of accountability via continued professional development (CPD), appraisal and personal development plans (PPD) at an individual level. The findings from Freeman and Walshe (2004), NAO (2003) and Hartley *et al.* (2002) work demonstrate that clinical governance has raised the profile of quality for NHS boards.

Braithwaite and Travaglia (2008) conclude that Boards and Executives participation is necessary to successfully embed clinical governance from the top of the organisation to grassroots in clinical and non-clinical areas.

In summary 'Clinical governance is also central to fashioning appropriate clinical care and organisational responsiveness. At the end of the day this is about working toward clinical and organisational excellence. No board or executive group should want to settle for anything less' (Braithwaite and Travaglia, 2008, p. 19).

Indeed no healthcare professional or manager could disagree with such a worthy aspiration. For us this captures the true essence of clinical governance.

Further work needs to be done in highlighting and embedding the importance of accountability at a team and individual level. This will only be achieved by having robust systems and processes in place that are adequately and appropriately resourced and managed.

Organisational structures

The NAO (2003) reported that the majority of NHS organisations have the necessary clinical governance foundations although these are not fully embedded in clinical directorates. 'Clinical governance is well established and embedded in the corporate systems of the vast majority of NHS Trusts, with board level executive and no non executive trust wide committee structures, and a strong executive function in the form of a clinical governance department or unit' (NAO 2003, p. 4). Wallace *et al.* (2004) like NAO (2003) highlighted the importance of having the necessary clinical governance systems and processes in place to ensure and improve quality. Similarly, Freeman and Walshe (2004) found that clinical governance 'structures seem to be well established' within the NHS Trusts surveyed. Braithwaite and Travaglia note the importance close relationship of clinical governance with corporate governance and the role of the boards in furthering clinical governance within their organisations. There is no doubt that without strong leadership and the appropriate organisational structures and accountabilities it is difficult to implement and embed effective clinical governance. However, we would argue that whilst the necessary structures are in place for the implementation of clinical governance, healthcare professionals and support staff need to be made aware of what these structures are, how they function and what benefits they provide to both the organisation and individual themselves. Furthermore, we would suggest that the development of any clinical governance systems and processes should involve and ultimately benefit patients, carers and the public they serve. Continuous quality improvement will not be achieved without having the necessary structures in place.

Continuous quality improvement

All the studies identified how clinical governance has influenced the quality improvement agenda. The NAO (2003) noted that there have been improvements in practice and patient care. However, this has been undertaken in an unsystematic and ad hoc manner and that requiring further attention and developments to ensure this becomes systematic in the future. Freeman and Walshe (2004) like NAO (2003) found that progress with quality improvement was less advanced than other aspects of clinical governance included in their study for instance corporate accountability and risk management. Wallace *et al.* (2004) reported improvements in patient care following the introduction of clinical governance by around 80% from the initial base line measure. This finding reinforces the need for advancing clinical governance frameworks within all NHS organisations. Degeling *et al.* (2003) unlike Freeman and Walshe (2004) and NAO (2003) evaluation studies which targeted organisational aspects of clinical governance focused on highlighting the impact of clinical governance reviews on practice. Six Welsh Trusts were involved where a combination of surveys and focus group interviews were undertaken to elicit healthcare staffs perspectives regarding clinical governance reviews. The study concluded that the impact of CHI reviews had minimal impact on the quality improvement agenda. Hartley *et al.*'s (2002) study of public health departments in the West Midland Region of England noted the positive effects of clinical governance surrounding CPD, appraisal and Life Long Learning and how these factors ultimately influence quality of care and services. Taking the empirical evidence provided by NAO (2003), Freeman and Walshe (2004), Wallace *et al.* (2004) and Degeling *et al.* (2003) into account it would be reasonable to suggests that clinical governance has played a major role in advancing and embedding the concept of continuously quality improvement within NHS organisations. Further work on engaging, empowering, enlightening and encouraging all staff working in clinical and non-clinical teams delivering patient care and services is essential. Braithwaite and Travaglia fully acknowledge the continuous quality improvement is a key element of clinical governance and consider it to be an umbrella term covering a range of activities including quality assurance, continuous education, planning and organising governance structure for safety and quality and the application standards, accreditation and encouraging clinical effectiveness.

As continuous quality improvement as reported by Freeman and Walshe (2004) has had a major impact on patient experience and patient outcome, we are in agreement with the authors of this report that further work to involve patients, users and the public is vital.

Performance management

Performance management emerges indirectly as a key feature of clinical governance in the way quality improvement is targeted and measured. The majority of these studies allude to the need for a systematic approach to performance management in order to detect changes both positive and negative with service and practice developments. Since the introduction of clinical governance within the NHS we have witnessed many improvements in health care with reductions in waiting times for elective procedures and outpatient appointments (DH 2005), improvements in treatments and outcomes, the adoption of evidence-based health care, improvements in clinical risk management and patient safety systems, the emergence of a open culture of learning, greater involvement of patients and the public in the planning, provision, delivery and evaluation of services. However, the evidence thus far is limited in confirming how these important changes with service provision have made a difference. The impact of clinical governance in our opinion has provided NHS boards of healthcare organisations, managers and healthcare professionals with a framework that has harmonised two seemingly contrasting concepts that of performance management and quality improvement. Performance management defined as 'the process of quantifying the efficiency and effectiveness of purposeful action and decision-making' (Waggoner *et al.* 1999) is an integral part of successful modernisation. This, according to McSherry and Pearce (2002), is because performance management involves developing, implementing and evaluating a series of complex systems and processes, which detect good and not-so-good practice of either devices or personnel. Taking Waggoner *et al.* (1999) and McSherry & Pearce (2002) evidence into account Garland (1998) argues that performance management is about the integration of various systems and sources of reported information in highlighting the overall quality status of the organisation. By combining Waggoner *et al.* (1999) and McSherry and Pearce (2002) works with the empirical study provided by Hartley *et al.* (2002) it is evident that Individual Performance Review (IPR) and Team Action Planning (TAP) play a fundamental role in achieving quality services within performance management frameworks. This is because successful implementation of clinical governance is dependent on the level of organisational, team and individual engagement with and in the various systems and processes. Performance management and continuous quality improvement collectively is about making and sustaining changes to improve the systems and processes which will ultimately impact on the patients outcomes. The concept of quality improvement is dear to the heart of most healthcare professionals because we all want the best for our patients and service users. Strange at it sounds to some the vast majority of healthcare managers also want to improve patient care and services. Yet, the empirical studies provided suggest that the development of robust systems and processes of continuous quality improvement and performance management is dependent on the organisational culture and working environment in which we work.

Culture

Culture emerges from the reported studies as a key contributor to the successful implementation and continued success of clinical governance. Returning to the DH (1997) original definition of clinical governance. 'a framework through which NHS organisations are accountable for continuously improving the quality of their services and safeguarding high standards of care by creating an environment in which clinical excellence will flourish' (DH 1997) is undoubtedly emerging as major framework for sustaining, assuring, developing and demonstrating excellence in practice. Based on the findings from the evaluation studies the creation of an environment in which clinical excellence will flourish is about creating and nurturing and open culture of learning and facilitation were CPD and Life Long Learning is valued and patients are placed at centre stage of all we do. The majority of the studies included in this brief literature review make either direct or indirect reference to organisational culture and change as major players in achieving successful governance. The NAO (2003) noted that there has been a change in clinical culture, which is becoming more transparent. Degeling *et al.* (2003) note that healthcare professionals have different experiences with understanding evaluations of clinical governance where each professional group seem to be influenced by its professional culture and efforts need to be made to increase awareness of how grass roots clinical staff perceive and evaluate clinical governance. To develop an organisational culture which values clinical governance several key factors emerge for its success.

Recipe for successes

The evidence to date suggests that to successfully develop a framework of clinical governance that ultimately impacts on the provision of excellence in practice is dependent on several factors:

- Strong leadership: leadership is required at all levels of the organisation resonating from the top of the organisation to staff working in all areas of the organisation. Where possible, the development of shared governance or self-governing teams should be nurtured in avoiding the stereotypical hierarchical approach to managing and leading change. Senior managers, clinicians and leaders of services need to lead by example and be committed for the course.
- Support and resources: from all staff working in the NHS and financial resourcing and backing needs to be provided in order to realise the full potential that clinical governance can provide. The various departments and associated systems and processes all need to communicate efficiently and effectively in order to realise the benefits of interdependency and collaborate working can provide.
- Culture: the creation of an honest, open and transparent culture where things go wrong or not so good are viewed in the light of a just blame culture where learning is at the heart of the organisation. This proactive as opposed to reactive approach to management and leadership is paramount to the successful implementation and continued development of clinical governance.
- CPD and Life Long Learning: Imperative to ensure that all staff have the necessary knowledge, skills and confidence to perform their role and responsibilities in a competent efficient and effective way. Lifelong learning should be seen as the norm where staff are willing to do things differently.

Conclusion

The empirical evidence to date reveals that the key critical success factors of clinical governance can be categories under five key areas: accountability, organisational structures, continuous quality improvement, performance management and culture. Despite these initial findings, much more empirical-based evaluation is needed to in order to confirm or repute the impact of clinical governance. A limitation of these studies is the fact that they are primarily focused on secondary care rather than in primary care or a combination of both. We would echo Halligan's (2006, p. 7) words 'what we have learnt, more than anything else, is that if clinical governances gains purchase in the hearts and minds of frontline staff and is built up from the bottom, then the strength of that frontline mandate is unstoppable'. The challenge is in acquiring the resource to engage frontline staff in taking ownership to continually drive clinical governance forward in their local context and setting.

Key points

- Dependent on your viewpoint clinical governance will be either embraced or resisted.
- The impact of clinical governance is emerging through the undertaking of empirical-based evaluation studies.
- Clinical governance has played a major role in highlighting and improving corporate accountability structures with NHS Trusts but more work needs to be done to ensure the same for individuals.
- The development of any clinical governance systems and processes should involve and ultimate benefit patients, carers and the public they serve.
- Performance management and continuous quality improvement collectively is about making and sustaining changes to improve the systems and processes which will ultimately impact on the patients outcomes.
- Based on the findings from the evaluation studies the creation of an environment in which clinical excellence will flourish is about creating and nurturing and open culture of learning and facilitation were CPD and Life Long Learning is valued and patients are placed at centre stage of all we do.

Suggested reading

Degeling, P., Maxwell, S., Kennedy, J., Coyle, B. & MacBeth, F. (2003) The impact of CHI: evidence from Wales. *Quality in Primary Care*, 11 (2) 147–154.

DH (1997) *The New NHS Modern Dependable*. The Stationery Office, London.

Freeman, T. & Walshe, K. (2004) Achieving progress through clinical governance? A national study of healthcare managers' perception in the NHS in England. *Quality and Safety in Healthcare*, 13, 335–343.

Hartley, M., Griffiths, R.K. & Saunders, K.L. (2002), An evaluation of clinical governance in the public health departments of the West Midlands Region. *Journal of Epidemiology and Community Health*, 56, 563–568.

National Audit Office (2003) *Achieving Improvements through Clinical Governance A Progress Report on Implementation by NHS Trusts*. National Audit Office, London.

Wallace, L.M., Boxall, M. & Spurgoen, P. (2004) Organisational change through clinical governance. *Clinical Governance: An Internal Journal*, 9 (1) 17–30.

References

Braithwaite, Y. & Travaglia (2008) An overview of clinical governance, policies, practices and initiatives. *Australian Health Review*, 32 (1) 10–22.

Degeling, P., Maxwell, S., Kennedy, J., Coyle, B. & MacBeth, F. (2003) The impact of CHI: evidence from Wales. *Quality in Primary Care*, 11 (2) 147–154.

DH (1997) *The New NHS Modern Dependable*. The Stationery Office, London.

DH (2010) Hospital Waiting Times and Waiting Lists, DH, London. Accessed 9 May 2010. http://www.dh.gov.uk/en/Publicationsandstatistics/Statistics/ Performancedataandstatistics/HospitalWaitingTimesandListStatistics/index.htm.

Freeman, T. & Walshe, K. (2004) Achieving progress through clinical governance? A national study of healthcare managers' perception in the NHS in England. *Quality and Safety in Healthcare*, 13, 335–343.

Gaminiara, E.J. (2000) *Book Review* of Clinical Governance: Making it Happen (eds M. Lugon & J. Secker-Walker). Royal Society of Medicine. *Quality in Health Care*, 9, 80.

Garland, G (1998) Governance Nursing Management, 56, 28–31.

Halligan, A. (2006) Clinical governance: assuring the sacred duty of trust to patients. *Clinical Governance: An International Journal*, 11 (1) 5–7.

Hartley, M., Griffiths, R.K. & Saunders, K.L. (2002) An evaluation of clinical governance in the public health departments of the West Midlands Region. *Journal of Epidemiology and Community Health*, 56, 563–568.

McSherry, R. & Pearce, P. (2002) *Clinical Governance: A Guide to Implementation for Health Care Professionals*. Blackwell Science, London.

National Audit Office (2003) *Achieving Improvements through Clinical Governance A Progress Report on Implementation by NHS Trusts*. National Audit Office, London.

Waggoner, D.B., Neeley, A.D. & Kennerley, N.P. (1999) The forces that shape organizational performance management systems:; an interdisciplinary view. *International Journal of Production Economics* 53 (60) 60–61.

Wallace, L.M., Boxall, M. & Spurgoen, P. (2004) Organisational change through clinical governance. Clinical Governance: *An International Journal*, 9 (1), 17–30.

Chapter 8

Education and Training for Clinical Governance

Rob McSherry and Paddy Pearce

Introduction

The chapter focuses on highlighting innovative and creative ways of introducing clinical governance into education and training departments of the National Health Service and Higher Education Institutes (HEIs) curricula in supporting Continued Professional Development (CPD) and Life Long Learning (LLL).

Clinical governance education and training within health care: turning myths into reality

Since the introduction of the term clinical governance (DH 1997) HEIs, healthcare organisations and individuals have firmly embraced the concept which has become an integral part of the continuous quality improvement agenda. To ensure that clinical governance continues to be the central framework for assuring quality, minimising risks, ensuring patient safety and public and professional confidence and experiences to name but a few, organisations and individuals have a major role and responsibility to ensure this happens. This will only occur by ensuring the concept is embraced and embedded within the HEIs educational curriculum and programmes and healthcare organisations education and training programmes. Furthermore, healthcare organisational objectives and development plans should be linked to CPD and LLL which is underpinned by clinical governance principles.

The remainder of this section provides examples of a clinical governance educational module for HEIs and a programme for healthcare organisations along with awareness raising for individuals.

Clinical Governance, third edition. By Rob McSherry and Paddy Pearce.
Published 2011 by Blackwell Publishing Ltd.

Teaching and learning clinical governance within higher educational institutions

Bayliss *et al.* (2001 p7) suggest that 'for the moderniszation of the NHS and successful implementation of clinical governance there must be a new curriculum, with new educational goals for the education of clinicians, managers and consumers'. The importance of clinical governance within health care as argued by Bayliss *et al.* (2001) has been recognised by HEIs leading to the development of several creative and innovative educational programmes, modules and workshops at both undergraduate and postgraduate levels. The intention of which is to ensure the students have a sound awareness of the key principles, components of clinical governance and its relevance to practice. Clinical governance as highlighted in chapters 2 and 4 should be part of everyone's roles, responsibilities forming part of an individual's professional accountability. Furthermore, such an approach aims to embed the concept of ongoing and continuous quality improvement as an integral part of an individual's day to day practice.

Whilst recognising the wide range and diverse educational requirements of individuals and acknowledging the variety of educational foundation, undergraduate and postgraduate health and social care programmes available. It is not our intention to offer a detailed educational programme but to provide an introduction and overarching framework that could be adopted/adapted to support your practice or individual requirements.

Theories of adult learning and clinical governance

Theories of adult learning and approaches are widely accessible and available in abundance in the guise of books, journal articles and e-learning materials/resources to name but a few. Adult learning theory or andragogy according to Knowles (1984, 1990) is bringing together the art and science in supporting adults to learn. An approach acknowledged by contemporary educational theorists Comings *et al.* (2008) and Sarkodie-Mensat (2000). Puliyel *et al.* (2006) cited in Craddock *et al.* (2006 p. 222) argue that adult learning 'is about the promotion of active learning grounded in the past experience of the learner and in the application of knowledge at a personal level'. The notion of promoting active learning informed by past and current experience is highly appropriate in informing and supporting individuals to learn about clinical governance.

Clinical governance as highlighted in chapters 2 and 3 is about learning from and sharing with other healthcare professionals both good and not so good experiences and practice in the furtherance of quality improvement and patient safety. Gosbee (1999) cited in Milligan (2007 p101) suggests that there 'is a risk that students can be de-motivated unless clear examples relevant to their practice are used when delivering human factor material' of which is highly relevant to clinical governance. Furthermore, Craddock *et al.* (2006) highlights the importance of Inter-professional education in supporting collaborative and partnership working to enhance learning. An approach that is essential when preparing, delivering and evaluating clinical governance education programmes.

> It is clear that the key challenge for curriculum developers of interprofessional educational initiatives lies in determining the most appropriate, theoretically sound, effective and locally responsive strategies for enabling successful health and social care inter-professioal collaboration (Craddock *et al.* 2006, p. 237).

Based on the works of Craddock *et al.* (2006) and Milligan (2007) when developing any clinical governance education and or training programme it is imperative to offer a sound balance between theory and examples from practice based on collaboration and partnership working approach.

Module learning outcomes

Cognitive and intellectual skills

- Integrate and synthesises the wider societal, political, professional and economical and cultural issues that may influence the utilisation of clinical governance both personally and organisationally.

Knowledge and understanding

- Demonstrate a comprehensive and critical understanding of the relevant theoretical and conceptual issues associated with the clinical governance framework.
- Demonstrate a systematic and critical understanding of the different component parts and how these interrelate within the clinical governance framework as applied to practice.

Practical/professional qualities and skills

- Autonomously interpret their own learning requirements relating to their current level of knowledge and practice regarding clinical governance.
- Apply new knowledge and critically evaluate the effectiveness of this on their practice at an individual, team and organisation level.

Key transferable

- Communicate and disseminate complex clinical governance information to solve problems in practice.

Module learning and teaching strategies

The module will be student lead using a combination of key lectures followed by seminars, workshops, case studies. The teaching and learning strategy will provide the students with the opportunity to explore a debate the relative merits and demerits of engaging with and applying the integrated governance framework to their practice. Case studies will be used to illustrate how clinical governance fits together. The students will be afforded the opportunity to use learning materials accessible via Virtual Learning Environment (VLE).

Indicative content

- Societal, political and professional drivers for clinical governance
- What is clinical governance?
- A guide to clinical governance
- Applying clinical governance in daily practice
- Identifying and exploring the barriers to the implementation of clinical governance
- Ethical and legal implications for clinical governance
- Identifying the impact of clinical governance
- The future implications of clinical governance

Module assessment

An individually written 5000-word assignment aimed at advancing clinical the governance framework. The student will have the opportunity to integrate and synthesise diverse knowledge, evidence and concepts in order to formulate new solutions and promote clinical governance within their practice. This is a 100% weighted assignment and should be submitted to the module leader at the end of the module.

Assessment criteria

- Rationale for the selection of the case study/scenario
- Comprehensive utilisations and critical understanding of the concepts and theory pertaining to clinical governance.

- Integration and synthesis of clinical governance issues, synthesis and conclusions.
- Application of clinical governance framework to practice setting.
- Utilisation of a wide range of sourced material to substantiate argument
- Presentation and referencing according to University guidelines.
  [All module learning outcomes assessed]

  **Essential Reading*
  **Recommended Reading*
  [*Incorporating books and journals]
  Additional Useful Information
  [Incorporating Websites]

Virtual learning environment (VLE)

In addition to tutor support, this module will be supported buy use of a blackboard site a Virtual Learning Environment]. The site will include lecture notes for each lecture that should be obtained prior to the lecture session taking place. In addition a discussion forum will be established to encourage debate and skills of critical reflection.

Tutorial and module support

The module leaders can be contacted to address any concerns or issues associated with the module. With reference to tutorial support, an initial group tutorial will be offered at the start of the module followed by personal tutorial support at the later stage.

Module evaluation

A series of structured evaluation will be taken at the outset and end of the module. The module team is always keen to receive feedback from the students at anytime throughout the course, which could contribute towards enhancing the quality of the module. At the end of the module the module team will undertake a formal evaluation using a structured questionnaires and group discussions.

We hope you enjoy the module and find the module booklet useful in guiding your learning.

Case study 8.1 provides an example of a potentially accredited university module that could be adapted/adopted to accommodate undergraduate/postgraduate level of study. The module could form part of a Degree/Masters programme.

Case study 8.1 Example of an undergraduate/postgraduate educational clinical governance module.

[This is intended as a guide for developing a module and not a comprehensive module/programme]

The 'Advancing practice using a clinical governance framework module' is designed to facilitate a systematic and critical understanding of the breadth and depth of clinical governance within health and social care setting. The emphasis of the module is on advancing practice using a clinical governance framework. The module considers the clinical, non-clinical and corporate aspects of clinical governance and how this can be influenced using the six key dimensions of governance: Clinical governance, corporate governance, information governance, research governance, financial governance and risk management. The student will be encouraged to critically reflect, synthesis and interpret how the use of the clinical governance framework may influence issues at the macro, micro and individual level. Assessment of the students learning will be undertaken using a case study based approach to resolve a clinical governance issue in practice.

Audience

The module could be targeted at undergraduate and postgraduate levels providing 20 academic credits running across an academic semester/term.

Module aims

- To facilitate the development of student's knowledge and awareness of the political, professional, economic and societal constructs surrounding clinical governance at both a personal and organisational level.
- To critically examine the theoretical/conceptual issues underpinning clinical governance.
- To develop a critical appreciation of relevant clinical governance tools, techniques and methods.
- To develop a critical appreciation of the relevance and impact of clinical governance both organisationally and individually.

Appendix 8.1
Clinical Governance Awareness Questionnaire

CLINICAL GOVERNANCE AWARENESS QUESTIONNAIRE

An addressed envelope is enclosed for you to return the questionnaire to ....

Your responses will confidential and no comment made would be attributable to you as an individual

Thank you in anticipation for completing and returning the questionnaire

In relation to the following questions, on a scale of one to five, one being strongly agree and five strongly disagree, please ✓ tick the box that matches your view most closely.

1. Clinical governance has a large part to play in improving patient care.

   Strongly Agree ☐☐☐☐☐ Strongly Disagree
   1 2 3 4 5

2. Clinical governance is part of my role and responsibility.

   Strongly Agree ☐☐☐☐☐ Strongly Disagree
   1 2 3 4 5

3. In using the clinical governance framework to support my practice I see benefit for myself.

   Strongly Agree ☐☐☐☐☐ Strongly Disagree
   1 2 3 4 5

4. Engaging with the clinical governance framework can influence patient care .

   Strongly Agree ☐☐☐☐☐ Strongly Disagree
   1 2 3 4 5

5. Clinical governance is a useful framework to change clinical practice at an individual, team and organisational level.

   Strongly Agree ☐☐☐☐☐ Strongly Disagree
   1 2 3 4 5

6. Engaging with the clinical governance framework can have a benefit in changing culture in the working environment.
7.

   Strongly Agree ☐☐☐☐☐ Strongly Disagree
   1 2 3 4 5

7. I have sufficient support and encouragement from peers and professionals to engage with the clinical governance framework.

Strongly Agree	1	2	3	4	5	Strongly Disagree

8. I have sufficient support from the management within my Directorate / clinical area to engage with clinical governance framework.

Strongly Agree	1	2	3	4	5	Strongly Disagree

9. In my training I received adequate information about what the clinical governance framework is and how it may aid improve quality services.

Strongly Agree	1	2	3	4	5	Strongly Disagree

10. I have a basic knowledge and understanding of clinical governance and associated systems and processes.

Strongly Agree	1	2	3	4	5	Strongly Disagree

11. I am confident to engage with the clinical governance framework.

Strongly Agree	1	2	3	4	5	Strongly Disagree

12. Have you had any clinical governance education or training?

Yes ☐1 No ☐2

13. If you answered yes to Question 12 above please specify

....
....
....
....

14. What do you feel are the main drivers for introducing clinical governance into the healthcare service? Please write these in the box provided.

15. What do you understand by the term clinical governance? Please write a short summary in the box below.

16. What would you describe as the key components of clinical governance? Please write these in the box provided.

17. Which of the following statements best describes clinical governance to you (✓ the appropriate box)

Clinical governance is the role and responsibility of chief executives and managers in maintaining quality care and services ☐1

Clinical governance is a quality framework and should be part of everyone's role and responsibility ☐2

Don't know ☐3

None of the above ☐4

18. Which of the following statements best describes the key components of clinical governance to you (✓ the appropriate box)

- Clinical governance is only about dealing with risks and managing complaints ☐1
- For clinical governance to occur in an organisation the following systems and processes need to be in place:
  - Risk management
  - Performance management
  - Quality improvement programme
  - Information
  - Accountability ☐2
- Don't know ☐3
- None of the above ☐4

19. Have you witnessed any change in practice that was related from individuals, teams or organisation engaging in the clinical governance framework?

Yes ☐1 No ☐2

20. If the answer to question 19 was 'yes' please provide details below.

....

....

....

21. Have you read any professional journal articles or books on clinical governance?

(1) Yes ☐[1]

(2) No ☐[2]

22. If the answer to question 21 was yes please indicate below which journal articles or books you read.

Journal Articles	**Books**

23. Can you list the three greatest barriers affecting your engagement with the clinical governance frameworks?

    1.

    2.

    3.

24. Please provide any necessary information relating to your answers or regarding to the questions contained in the questionnaire in the box provided.

    Please identify the question/s your comments relate to

Please tick the appropriate boxes and add any comments in the space provided.

25. What is your position?

Doctor	☐ 1
Hospital Midwife	☐ 2
Community Midwife	☐ 3
Registered Nurse	☐ 4
Student Nurse Diploma Pathway	☐ 5
Student Nurse Diploma Year 1	☐ 6
Student Nurse Diploma Year 2	☐ 7
Student Nurse Diploma Year 3	☐ 8
Student Nurse Degree Pathway	☐ 9
Student Nurse Degree Year 1	☐ 10
Student Nurse Degree Year 2	☐ 11
Student Nurse Degree Year 3	☐ 12

Allied Health Professional
(please state)..

26.When did you qualify as a Healthcare Professional?

27. Please state your grade:

28. Please state which clinical speciality you currently work in:

29. Which of the following hours do you work?

10-14	☐ 1
15-20	☐ 2
21-24	☐ 3
25-30	☐ 4
31-37.5	☐ 5

30. Please state your professional qualifications and additional qualifications.

Professional:

Additional:

Thank you very much
for taking the time to complete and
return this questionnaire.
All your responses will be confidential
and no comment will attributable to you
as an individual.

Clinical governance education and training within healthcare organisations

The education and training needs of healthcare staff should be provided at three levels within a local healthcare organisation where the information about clinical governance is designed with a specific targeted audience in mind Table 8.1.

Table 8.1 highlights how the employer should seek to establish the educational needs of their employees, perhaps through the development and implementation of a staff 'clinical governance awareness questionnaire detailed in appendices 8.1'. Furthermore, the education and training programme(s) should be designed to best suit the target audience, as highlighted in Fig. 8.1.

Figure 8.1 demonstrates the links between the various structures of the NHS and the need for education and training on clinical governance. It is imperative that all levels of the NHS are aware of their educational responsibilities in informing and educating their staff about the what,

Table 8.1 Targeting clinical governance education and training with an organisation.

Target audience	Rational
Organisational	At an organisational level all new employees of the Trust should attend the induction programme where a presentation on clinical governance should be given, associated with an overview of the structures and processes linked to clinical governance.
Team/directorate	At a team/directorate level a specific education and training programme could be delivered via the 'rolling development programmes' where clinical governance is aligned to the specific activities of the team. Case studies, critical reflections and reviews of complaints are used as examples of where clinical governance fits in with practice, accompanied by networking and sharing good and not so good practices within the teams and organisations and where necessary externally to other organisations.
Individual	At an individual level the education and training needs of the individual should be associated with learning needs established after the performance review, forming the basis of the personal development plan linked to the AfC and KSF. These could be attendance on programme, modules and course, seminars or workshops.

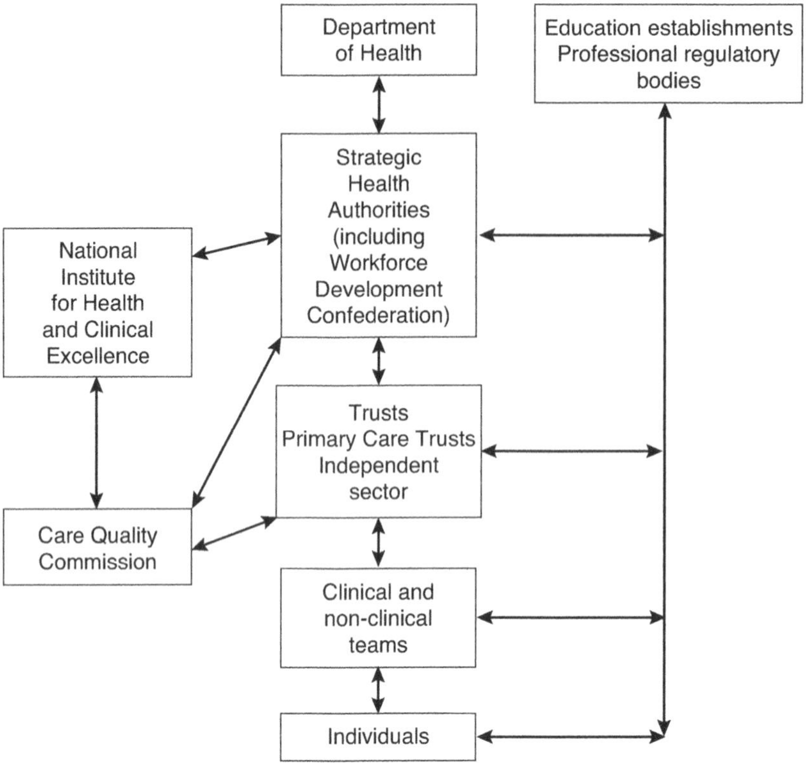

Fig. 8.1 The NHS structures that require clinical governance educational awareness sessions.

why and how of clinical governance can make a difference to and for people.

The National Institute for Clinical Excellence and Health (NICE) also have a responsibility to inform staff of the new guidelines to practice in keeping with the philosophy of clinical governance. Similarly, the Care Quality Commission (which replaced by The Healthcare Commission and prior to this the Commission for Health Improvements (CHI)) have a responsibility for reviewing the effectiveness of clinical governance arrangements for all NHS Trusts & PCTs, in the course of which the provision and effectiveness of education and training may be assessed. The most difficult aspect in the education and training of clinical governance, we believe, is in linking it to the organisation, teams and individuals and in releasing personnel from their daily clinical duties to attend clinical governance education courses, etc. (Phipps 2000). For this to be effective the NHS organisations boards need to be committed and supportive with both monetary and resources to enable and empower staff to embrace governance to be practiced (Bevinton *et al.* 2004). Therefore the development of education and training session that focuses on knowledge and awareness about clinical governance is imperative.

Knowledge and awareness raising of clinical governance

All NHS employees should be made aware of the idea that for clinical governance to become a reality, it is everybody's business. Clinical governance will only become a reality by engaging and using its frameworks. To make certain that clinical governance becomes known and owned by all NHS staff, educational and training programmes need to be directed to the appropriate audiences as highlighted in Table 8.1. The targeted educational and training programmes on clinical governance need to cover the key components such as risk management, performance management, quality improvement, information and communication, accountability, patient and public involvement. Furthermore, the utilisation of relevant examples and case studies taken from real life situations to reinforce understanding and the relevance of clinical practice to their own practice is essential.

The development of any educational and training programme for teams or individuals should be linked to demands of the local organisation or educational requirement highlighted via the Strategic Health Authorities Workforce Departments.

Case study 8.2 Clinical governance education and training within healthcare organisations.

Any devised educational and training programmes should be:

- *Multiprofessional* – applicable and relevant to all healthcare professionals
- *Collaborative in nature* – highlighting the importance of integrated team working, pathways of care and patient journeys/experience/stories.
- *Practically focused* – reflect real life situations along with the culture and working environment of the organisation.
- *Evidence based* – be supported by relevant guidelines and research.
- *Utilising a variety of teaching and learning methods* – incorporate a combination of lectures, workshops, seminars, case studies to enlighten, encourage individual participation, engagement and debates.
- *Competency based* – linked to the AfC, KSF frameworks and risk management training.
- *Evaluated regularly* – to receive feedback from participants and speakers to inform and enhance the quality of the programme.
- *Accreditable* – could be accredited by local Universities.

An example of a proposed healthcare organisations educational and training programme or framework for clinical governance is highlighted in Box 8.1.

Box 8.1 Aim: To provide an introduction to clinical governance.

Learning outcomes:

- To describe what is meant by clinical governance
- To describe the key processes and components of clinical governance
- To describe what clinical governance means in relation to individual practice
- To apply the concept of clinical governance to clinical case studies identified from practice
- To locate evidence and sources of information on clinical governance
- To evaluate the effectiveness of the course on the individual's understanding of clinical governance in relation to their practice.

All clinical governance educational and training programmes should be about learning from the practical experience gained in the workplace, with the learning shared and disseminated across multiprofessional boundaries. This approach to shared and problem based learning is more likely to be successful, an approach advocated by the following statements:

> Learning in teams, developing multidisciplinary education and training across different agencies, is the way forward for creating learning environments. It will encourage healthcare professionals to work in partnerships in sharing ideas and solving problems that focus on what is important for patients. (Squire 2000, p. 1015)

> New approaches to undergraduate medical education, such as the introduction of problem based learning, joint education with other professional disciplines, should in time improve team working skills; the importance of team working has been emphasised by the General Medical Council. (DH 2004b, p. 65.). The success of any healthcare organisations education and training programme is dependent on the engagement and integration of the individual and how they view and regard clinical governance.

Individual awareness of clinical governance

The employee should make known through their individual personal development plans need to reflect the AfC requirements (DH 2004a and 2004b) and be linked to the KSF (DH 2005) for their job profile. This process will ensure relevant training needs and competences are developed in a systematic and logical way commensurate with the clinical governance frameworks. The barrier for some organisations, teams and individuals is in establishing what they need to know, i.e. where clinical governance relates to them and their practices and in accessing the information on clinical governance. This is where having knowledge and understanding of clinical governance is essential if it is to become an integral part of healthcare professions' daily practice and not seen to be another obstacle to practice.

Conclusion

Likewise local universities providing healthcare courses need to develop clinical governance modules to educate both their pre and post registration healthcare students about clinical governance.

Key points

- Organisations and individuals have firmly embraced the concept which has become an integral part of continuous quality improvement agenda.
- Clinical governance should be part of everyone's roles, responsibilities forming part of an individual's professional accountability.
- The education and training needs of healthcare staff should be provided at three levels within a local healthcare organisation where the information about clinical governance is designed with a specific targeted audience in mind.
- Clinical governance will only become a reality by engaging and using its frameworks.
- The development of any educational and training programme for teams or individuals should be linked to demands of the local organisation or educational requirement highlighted via the Strategic Health Authorities Workforce Departments.
- All clinical governance educational and training programmes should be about learning from the practical experience gained in the workplace, with the learning shared and disseminated across multiprofessional boundaries.
- The success of any healthcare organisations education and training programme is dependent on the engagement and integration of the individual and how they view and regard clinical governance.

Suggested reading

Craddock, D., O'Halloran, C., Borthwick, A. & McPherson, K. (2006) Interprofessional education in health and social care: fashion or informed practice? *Learning in Health and Social Care* 5 (4) 220–242.

Milligan, F.J. (2007) Establishing a culture for patient safety: the role if education. *Nurse Education Today* 27, 95–102.

References

Bayliss, P., Hill, P., Calman, K. & Hamilton, J. (2001) Evaluation for clinical governance. *The British Journal of Clinical Governance*, 6 (1) 7–8.

Bevinton, J., Halligan, A. & Cullun, R. (2004) Understanding organisations: Part 2 Hospital Doctor 8July.

Comings, J., Garner, B. & Smith, C. eds (2008) *Review of Adult Learning and Literacy Volume 4: Connecting Research, Policy, and Practice*. Taylor and Francis e-library, New Jersey, USA.

Craddock, D., O'Halloran, C., Borthwick, A. & McPherson, K. (2006) Interprofessional education in health and social care: fashion or informed practice? *Learning in Health and Social Care*, 5 (4) 220–242.

Department of Health (1997) *The New NHS, Modern Dependable*, DH, London.

Department of Health (2004a) *Agenda for Change – What Will It Mean for You?* A guide for staff. DH, London.

Department of Health (2004b) *The Knowledge and Skills Framework (NHS KSF) and Development Review Process (October 2004)*. DH, London.

Gosbee, J.W. (1999) Human factors engineering is the basis for a practical error in medicine curriculum Center for Medical Informatics, Mitchigan Sate University. http://www.dcs.gla.ac.uk/˜johnson/papers/HECS_99/Gosbee.htm. Accessed 08 December 2009.

Knowles, M.S. (1984) *Andragogy in Action: Applying Modern Principles of Adult Learning*. Jossey-Bass, San Francisco.

Knowles, M.S. (1990) *The Adult Learner: A Neglected Species*. Gulf Publishing, Houston, TX.

Milligan, F.J. (2007) Establishing a culture for patient safety: the role of education. *Nurse Education Today*, 27, 95–102.

Phipps, K. (2000) Nursing and clinical governance. *British Journal of Clinical Governance*, 5 (2) 69–70.

Puliyel, M.M., Puliyel, J.M. & Puliyel, U. (1999) Drawing on adult learning theory to teach personal and professional values. *Medical Teacher*, 21, 513–515. Cited in Craddock, D., O'Halloran, C., Borthwick, A. & McPherson, K. (2006) Interprofessional education in health and social care: fashion or informed practice? *Learning in Health and Social Care*, 5 (4) 220–242.

Sarkodie-Mensat, K. ed (2000) *Reference Services for the Adult Learner: Challenging Issues for the Traditional and Technical Era*. The Howard Press Information Press, New York, USA.

Squire, S. (2000) Clinical governance in action: Part 7: effective learning. *Professional Nurse*, 16 (4) 1014–1015.

Chapter 9

Conclusion: The Future of Clinical Governance for Healthcare Professionals

Rob McSherry and Paddy Pearce

In this third edition we have described why clinical governance was needed and what it is, together with its key components and how they relate to practicing clinicians, teams and organisations. Furthermore we have tried to illustrate the impact of clinical governance along with highlighting the importance within the education and training settings.

The challenge for some healthcare organisations, teams and individuals according to Halligan (2006) remain in resolving the barriers, keeping abreast with current healthcare reform and policy, which does affect the successful implementation of clinical governance. For example the current financial deficit facing NHS organisation, has lead to job cuts and service reviews. We believe these changes have affected staff moral and may ultimately have a direct and detrimental effect on patient experience and continuous quality improvement making it imperative for individual, teams and organisations to keeping up to date with the law as outlined in Chapter 6.

Given the importance with which the current government and no doubt future governments continue to regard clinical governance, it goes without saying that it remains here to stay. Some authors would argue '*Integrated Governance*' should replace that of clinical governance. We would echo the desire for integrated governance as the next evolutionary stage of development for governance in health and social care settings. This approach would acknowledge the inter-dependency of the various faces of governance in integrating the various components of governance for example, corporate, clinical, research, information and financial. Integrated governance according DH (2006 p. 10) is defined as

---

Clinical Governance, third edition. By Rob McSherry and Paddy Pearce.
Published 2011 by Blackwell Publishing Ltd.

> systems, processes and behaviours by which trusts lead, direct and control their functions in order to achieve organisational objectives, safety and quality of service and in which they relate to patients and carers, the wider community and partner organisations

The DH (2006) definition along with the integrated governance handbook is primarily aimed at executive and non-executive NHS board members and has not transcended to the frontline staff. We acknowledge the inclusivity of integrated governance and endorse its underlying principles and aspiration as the way forward for quality improvement, patient and staff safety along with patient, public and staff experience as collect umbrella term for governance. However, we believe that clinical governance should remain independent but an integral part of the integrated governance framework because it is a concept or set of systems and processes that clinicians and managers have embraced and recognise.

To shift the focus of clinical governance away to that of integrated governance too quickly may ultimately have a detrimental effect on healthcare staff's perceptions of governance and lead to disengagement rather than continuing to engage with the term in the future.

In the past year or so the term clinical governance has become less commonly used. The DH and others have changed the language and it would appear that some of the key components of clinical governance have been re-badged as 'Patient Safety', whilst we would whole heartedly agree that patient safety should be at the forefront of all healthcare organisations and their employees. Such an approach may lead to isolated initiatives that may not fully consider the interdependency of the key components of the clinical governance framework. Such an approach could be conceived as a retrograde step. Throughout this book we have attempted to emphasise the importance of holistic and collaborative shared partnership working within and between organisations and the interdependency of all the clinical and non-clinical component of governance. For us the key to progress is genuine collaboration and the recognition that by working together we can improve patient experience and outcomes and offer a truly integrated governance approach in the future. As espoused by Heath (1998) effective integrated working is dependent on having strong seams within and between the component parts

> the team is a structure made up of distinct components, each of different materials. If the patient is to be offered a coherent service, there must be obvious seams between each area of skill, with sufficient overlap to ensure that the whole holds together.

The desire of the healthcare professionals and public alike for seamless continuous improvement in clinical quality, in striving for excellence, further reinforces the need for clinical governance. Over the past 62 years we have witnessed many changes in the NHS, where some seem to have introduced a term 'changing things for the sake of change'. The changes attributed to clinical governance are somewhat different and cannot be viewed by the cynics as alluded to by Baker (2000) – the change for changing sake approach to healthcare policy – because clinical governance is a broad framework that has encompassed many different strands of quality under a collective umbrella and made leaders of healthcare organisations responsible and accountable for assuring clinical and non-clinical quality. Whilst the NHS is in difficult and challanging times clinical governance provide continuous NHS organisations, teams and individuals with a golden opportunity to make genuine and lasting improvements in the systems and process of care delivery as managerial and clinical responsibilities are harmonised. Clinical governance principles need to be aligned to support undivided teams and organisation to achieve the quality, innovation, prevention and productivity (QIPP) agenda.

The real opportunities and challenges facing some healthcare organisations, teams and individuals are in the development of realistic and achievable strategies that support their quest for the continuous quality improvement in providing excellent clinical care. Organisations, teams and individuals that are truly committed to clinical governance will realise that clinical governance is everybody's business, by ensuring a multidisciplinary and multiagency approach to the development of future services. For clinical governance to realise its potential the concept as part of the AfC should be written into all job descriptions and contracts of employment for all NHS employees, an approach that reinforces the concept of ensuring accountability by all NHS staff for the provision of high quality care. Clinical governance must be included in the induction of all employees in ensuring a move towards the development, implementation and evaluation of the care, treatment or interventions they provide. A culture of openness, honesty and transparency with a willingness to learn from mistakes and share good and not so practices needs to become the norm. The creation of such culture continues to require time, commitment, vision, ambition and patience over a long period, where good communications, collaborations and partnerships between and within the systems and processes akin to clinical governance, along with the professions, are fundamental (Donaldson 2000).

The challenge for the future of healthcare organisations, teams and individuals is in resolving the barriers to clinical governance, barriers that are related to the founding principles of the NHS in ensuring universal access to a comprehensive service based on clinical need where equity, diversity and equality of the services will be assured for all. These principles can only be assured in an organisation that is open to criticism and learns from its mistakes, as the recent media attention continues to inform the NHS. To ensure this open culture where expressing one's concerns or celebrating success becomes the norm, management and leadership that is transformational and democratic in nature requires development, where staff are valued and developed through the instigation of mutual partnerships, shared decision-making and ownership that reinforces the concept of accountability via the clinical governance framework. The task for individual healthcare professionals is in developing their knowledge, understanding and skills of applying the concept of clinical governance to their daily practice. Aligning clinical governance alongside their personal and professional development plans and KSF can only serve the professional well in the future. However, this will only become effective in an organisation that proactively seeks and values the true potential that clinical governance can unlock for their own organisation. Genuine sustained support and commitment needs to be guaranteed from the boards to the shop floor. The National Plan 2000 clearly stated and stipulated the need for the adoption of a clinical governance framework by the organisation, team and individual by basing the entire document around assuring the continuous quality improvements of the NHS – a quality service that will be measured and evaluated against set national standards of care derived from the best available evidence published by NICE. The adherence to these standards along with the implementation of the clinical governance framework that are continuously assessed and reviewed by CQC, which should be viewed as a supporting not a policing agency in evolving the future of the NHS.

We believe that as healthcare professionals concerned with providing the best standards of care to our patients, carers, service users and the public we need to continually embrace this wonderful opportunity to partake in the reformation of our NHS. Clinical governance within an 'Integrated Governance' framework remains a vehicle to enable us to do this efficiently and effectively. So let us get involved with clinical governance in making a real and lasting difference for our NHS and all patients in our care.

Good luck!

References

Baker, M. (2000) *Making Sense of the NHS White Papers*, 2nd edn. Radcliffe Medical Press Ltd, Oxford.

Department of health (2006) *Integrated Governance Handbook: A Handbook for Executives and Non-executives in Healthcare Organisations*. HMSO, London.

Donaldson, L.J. (2000) Clinical governance; a mission to improve. *British Journal of Clinical Governance*, 5 (1) 6–8.

Halligan, A. (2006) Real reform of health service 'a deceit'. In: *Financial Times* (ed. N. Timmins) 3rd April. http://news.ft.com/cms/s/7e5498ba/c2ae/11da-ac03-00079e2340.html.

Heath, I. (1998) A Seamless service. BMJ, 317, 1723–1724.

Index

ᑫ/P

9 781444 331110